"Boakye, Mwale and colleagues shine a much needed light on the current limitations and health inequalities of clinical neuropsychology in the UK serving an increasingly diverse population in terms of ethnicity and culture."

Katherine Carpenter, *Consultant Clinical Neuropsychologist and President of The British Psychological Society 2021-22*

"This book adjoins the 'socio-politico-cultural' context to biopsychosocial neuropsychological formulation, adding absolutely essential understanding of the patient experience and influences on outcomes in neurorehabilitation."

Dr Gerald ('Jerry') Burgess, *Director of Clinical Neuropsychology Programmes, Salomons Institute for Applied Psychology; SPANS-X author*

"Having vast years of senior nursing experience in neurorehabilitation, the systemic approaches in this book encompassing a culturally diverse cohort of clients provides not only a tool but a 'stop and challenge own bias moment' for the whole multidisciplinary team. Barriers of neuropsychology are explored, and these deliberately challenge the status quo."

Dee Kapfunde, *Divisional Director of Nursing & Governance, Children's, Women's, Diagnostics, Therapies, Outpatients, Pharmacy, Critical Care. St George's University Hospitals, NHS Foundation Trust*

"It presents an alternative discourse on disability and disadvantage in neurorehabilitation, challenging us to develop culturally sensitive practices that lead to meaningful person-centred change. It draws on the growing literature on diversity and inclusion, with experts in the field offering thoughtful, compassionate and pragmatic recommendations for culturally informed assessment, formulation and intervention."

Dr Noelle Blake, *Consultant Clinical Neuropsychologist and Teaching Fellow, University of Surrey*

I0028283

Systemic Approaches to Brain Injury Treatment

This book is an exploration of key systemic and socio-political considerations when working with people whose lives have been impacted by neurological injury and with those who care for them.

Expert contributors consider the impact of intersectionality across domains that include gender, sexuality, class, education, religion and spirituality, race, culture, and ability/disability. It offers relevant literature in the field of neuropsychology as well as clinical case studies that provide inspiration and key reflections for clinicians, neurological specialist therapists, and medical staff alike. Chapters discuss navigating intersectionality in couple therapy, hidden social inequalities in paediatric neurorehabilitation, racial microaggression in inpatient settings, and more.

This book is essential for all health and social-care practitioners working in the field of brain injury and chronic illness who want to challenge the status quo and advocate for diversity and inclusion.

Dr. Ndidi Boakye is Head of Neuropsychology and Clinical Health (Croydon NHS Trust) and Director of The Psych Practice Limited (an independent psychology and rehabilitation service). Dr. Boakye is a Consultant Clinical Neuropsychologist, Couple Therapist, and lecturer with extensive experience across multiple settings. Her interests involve using systemic and critical psychology approaches in neurorehabilitation, long-term conditions, couple/family work, teams, and organisations.

Dr. Amanda Mwale is a UK clinical psychologist with experience working across clinical health settings, including neurorehabilitation. She has a special interest in systemic practices, including working in collaboration with a diverse workforce. She is also committed to staff support and well-being in teams and organisations. She co-authored the book, *Becoming a Clinical Psychologist: Everything You Need to Know.*

Systemic Approaches to Brain Injury Treatment

Navigating Contemporary Practice

**Edited by Ndidi Boakye and
Amanda Mwale**

Routledge
Taylor & Francis Group

NEW YORK AND LONDON

Designed cover image: Cover art by clinpsych_ind

First published 2023
by Routledge
605 Third Avenue, New York, NY 10158

and by Routledge
4 Park Square, Milton Park, Abingdon, Oxon, OX14 4RN

Routledge is an imprint of the Taylor & Francis Group, an informa business

Library of Congress Cataloging-in-Publication Data
A catalog record for this title has been requested

ISBN: 9781032314495 (hbk)
ISBN: 9781032314501 (pbk)
ISBN: 9781003309819 (ebk)

DOI: 10.4324/9781003309819

Typeset in Times New Roman
by codeMantra

Contents

Acknowledgements

Firstly, this book would not have been possible without the lived stories and experiences of individuals, families, and communities from minoritised groups living with brain injury. We thank and salute you for your bravery in sharing your stories. As people of faith, we thank God for the privilege and opportunity to serve these communities and hope that this book goes some way in breaking barriers and pushing conversations further to bring about the necessary change that will mean better health outcomes for all.

We are eternally grateful to our families and friends who have supported us along the way, encouraging us and cheering us on whist we (and they) also experienced some of the challenges discussed in this book.

I (Ndidi) thank my mother for believing in me and instilling values that have shaped me to be the psychologist I am today. I still recall the day when one of my undergraduate lecturers told me that people like me don't become psychologists, and you said I could be anything I wanted to be in this world and that only God had the final say in my life – thank you. I'm grateful to you and Daddy for raising me with strong Christian values and ensuring my identity was robust. My knowledge of who I am as a person carried me through the many knocks I experienced in this profession, enabling each blow to be a stepping-stone to where I am today – thank you.

I thank my husband – my favourite cheerleader and champion. Your unfailing love and dedication meant you listened, nurtured, encouraged, and entertained the ideas that led to me undertaking this process – thank you. I love and cherish you so dearly.

I thank my wonderful siblings (including the ones I inherited via law) for their unwavering support. Ngozi, thank you for helping me articulate racial microaggressions so well. I appreciate you very much. I thank my cousins, uncles, aunties, and mother-in-law. Thank you all for believing in me and being so proud of me. This book is dedicated to you with all my love.

I (Amanda) would like to thank every person who is dear to me for all of their love, kindness, and support. In keeping with the metaphor of the Tree of Life, I am very blessed to have so many "leaves" that represent colleagues, mentors, teachers of life, relatives, friends, and confidants. You have all shaped me and my values, particularly in relation to courage and social justice. Thank you for providing me with safe spaces to be the woman and psychologist I am continuing to become. A special thank you to my mother, brother, cousin, and partner, who all have been so encouraging and excited about this book. It's finally here! Thank you for believing in me and being so proud of me.

Thank you to Indiana Montaque [@clinpsych_ind] for gifting us with an amazing cover. We appreciate your generosity so much – thank you.

A very special thanks to the following individuals for all their support in the process:

Ghayda Javed, Laura Bach, Adela Curaj, Ngozi Ebubedike, Meiron Yusuf-George, Noelle Blake, Jonathan Edwards and his team, Francesca Curtis, Morvwen Duncan, Jonathan Davidson, David Frederick, Katherine Carpenter, Jenny Altschulter, Fergus Gracey, Giles Yeates, and every supervisor who we have had along this journey.

Contributors

Dr. Rob Agnew (he/him) (ORCID: 0000–0002-3105-2984) is a clinical psychologist with a background in neurorehabilitation, autism, challenging behaviour, and complex/differential diagnosis. He lectures in several London universities on LGBTQ+ issues and research and is a committee member of the British Psychological Society's Section of Sexuality. He is a gay, cisgendered, White male and an ally of the trans community.

Dr. Shabnam Berry-Khan (ORCID: 0000–0002-5740-4132) is owner of PsychWorks Associates Ltd., a diverse case management and treating psychology service working with personal injury clients. She has developed a unique model that brings individuals' needs to the core of the meanings around rehabilitation. It speaks to authentic experiences, closing an important gap in inclusive rehabilitation within the personal injury field.

Dr. Ndidi Boakye (ORCID: 0000–0003-4066–0970) is Head of Neuropsychology and Clinical Health (Croydon NHS Trust) and Director of The Psych Practice Limited (an independent psychology & rehabilitation service). Dr Boakye is a Consultant Clinical Neuropsychologist, Couple Therapist, and lecturer with extensive experience across multiple settings. Her interests involve using systemic and critical psychology approaches in neurorehabilitation, long-term conditions, couple/family work, teams, and organisations.

Dr. Sue Copstick (ORCID: 0000–0002-5875-3879) is a Consultant Clinical Neuropsychologist and Honorary Senior Lecturer at Glasgow University. She has spent 25 years in NHS Neuroscience Centres in Glasgow and Plymouth, providing assessment and treatments for Neurosurgical and Neurological conditions. She was Clinical Director of the Disabilities Trust until 2021 and currently works in Neurological Rehabilitation in London with HighView Care Services.

Dr. Gemma Costello (ORCID: 0000–0002-6425-5796) is a specialist educational psychologist in paediatric neuropsychology. She is the Head of Psychosocial Services at The Children's Trust, working as part of an inter-disciplinary team supporting children, young people, and their families following acquired brain injury. Gemma is committed to promoting educational psychology in paediatric acquired brain injury and contributing to educational and neuropsychology training.

Dr. Sheeba Ehsan (ORCID: 0000–0001-5259–7206) has over 20 years of clinical experience in neurosciences and neuropsychology. Her collaborations have led to key papers in high-impact journals. She has a keen interest in cross-cultural test adaptation across clinical procedures (fMRI, Awake craniotomy, WADA test). She practices both within the NHS and the private sector. Her work has often focused on supporting marginalised groups.

Dr. Fergus Gracey (ORCID: 0000–0002-1416–7894) is a Senior Research Fellow at the University of East Anglia in the Department of Clinical Psychology, seconded from his post as Consultant Clinical Neuropsychologist in Cambridgeshire Community Services (NHS) Trust. He was formerly the Clinical Lead for the Cambridge Centre for Paediatric Neuropsychological Rehabilitation. His clinical and research interests are in neuropsychological rehabilitation, specifically self-regulation, identity, emotional adjustment, and psychological therapy following brain injury. Dr. Gracey holds honorary positions as a Consultant Clinical Neuropsychologist with the Cambridge Centre for Paediatric Neuropsychological Rehabilitation and NIHR CLAHRC East of England, is a member of the Board of Associate Editors of *Neuropsychological Rehabilitation*, is a member of the Board of Trustees for Headway Cambridgeshire, and is a Clinical Associate at the MRC Cognition and Brain Sciences Unit, Cambridge.

Dr. Lorraine Haye (ORCID: 0000–0002-7973-1900), Kaizen Psychology Ltd, is a clinical psychologist with experience working in Neuropsychology and long-term health conditions across the full care pathway. She completed her post-qualification Neuropsychology training at the University of Glasgow. She currently works in community neurorehabilitation and is a director of a psychology practice providing services for children, adults, families, and organisations.

Dr. Jenny Jim (ORCID: 0000–0002-6788–8759), Consultant clinical psychologist, Psychology Lead at The Children's Trust, and honorary professor and lecturer is an award-winning professional (British Medical Association, 2018 – User Engagement; British Psychological Society's DoN Early Career Award, 2020). She is the lead editor of the book *Psychological Therapy for Paediatric Acquired Brain Injury: Innovations for Children, Young People, and Families*, Routledge (2020).

Dr. Camille Julien (ORCID: 0000–0002-9510-7155) is a Consultant clinical neuropsychologist and community neurorehabilitation lead at

Kings College Hospital and Homerton Healthcare NHS Foundation Trusts. She is interested in systemic models of practice for team work, service design, delivery, and the cognitive and psychosocial consequences of living with acquired brain injury. She set up psychology provision for the UK's first MDT aphasia programme.

Dr. Valéria Lowing (ORCID: 0000–0001-5510–8068) is a Clinical Psychologist at The Children's Trust and author. Her work focuses primarily on children, young people neurorehabilitation, and parents' mental health. She has developed mental health courses and workshops for children and adults. Valéria is an award-winning Clinical Psychologist for representing Psychology within her community and creating viable ways for those in need to access adequate support.

Dr. Amanda Mobley (ORCID: 0000–0002-5450-1180) is a Consultant Clinical Neuropsychologist working in the NHS and in independent practice. She is also the Co-Director of The Brain Place. Dr. Mobley is actively involved in a number of professional appointments, including the Motor Neurone Disease Association and West Mental Strategic Clinical Network for Parkinson's Disease. She is also an Associate Lecturer at various universities.

Dr. Amanda Mwale (ORCID: 0000–0001-5251–8862) is a UK clinical psychologist with experience working across clinical health settings, including neurorehabilitation. She has a special interest in systemic practices, including working in collaboration with a diverse workforce. She is also committed to staff support and well-being in teams and organisations. She co-authored the book, *Becoming a Clinical Psychologist: Everything You Need to Know.*

Steve Nash is a senior social worker at The Children's Trust who believes in promoting the rights and advocacy of CYPF affected by ABI. Steve is committed to participation and young people having a voice in the organisation, and he regularly facilitates groups with service users to establish their views and thoughts as to the development of our work.

Dr. Alison Perkins (ORCID: 0000–0003-0324–365X) is a clinical psychologist practicing within the multidisciplinary team at The Children's Trust, which provides neurorehabilitation for children with brain injury. She has a particular interest in the impact of an ABI on the young person's developing identity and the sociocultural factors that influence this.

Dr. Masuma Rahim (ORCID: 0000–0002-7880–9737), Barts Health NHS Trust, is a clinical psychologist, neuropsychologist, and systemic practitioner. She works in community neurorehabilitation and in independent practice.

Dr. Carol Sampson (ORCID: 0000–0001-5831-1141) is a consultant clinical neuropsychologist with over 25 years' experience in the NHS developing community neuropsychology rehabilitation services. In 2019 Carol established Integrity Neuropsychology Services (INSneuro) CIC, a social enterprise organisation, to make neuropsychological approaches more accessible to people from disadvantaged communities. Carol is passionate about workforce development and increasing access and diversity within the neuropsychology workforce.

Chezelle Scholes (ORCID: 0000–0002-0663–5491) is a social worker at The Children's Trust with experience in safeguarding teams in the Local Authority and an interest in brain injuries and contextual safeguarding in her current role. Chezelle recently contributed to the development of national guidance for social workers in supporting children and young people post ABI.

Dr. Eva Sundin (ORCID: 0000–0001-7490-035X) is a professor in psychology at Nottingham Trent University, where she has been employed since 2006. She received her PhD in Applied Psychology from Umea University in 1994. She has been a practising clinical psychologist and accredited cognitive behavioural therapist. Currently, she works with the Motor Neurone Disease Association to raise awareness about Motor Neurone Diseases.

Dr. Penny Trayner (ORCID: 0000–0002-2992-0287) is a paediatric clinical neuropsychologist and founder of a community-based rehabilitation service in Manchester, UK. She is an Honorary Lecturer at the University of Manchester and creator of Goal Manager®, an award-winning rehabilitation goal-planning platform. Penny is also a professional DJ and has used her skills to co-design the 'Brains Powered by Music' DJing for rehabilitation programme.

Dr. Claire F. Whitelock (ORCID: 0000–0001-5191–517X) is a Clinical Psychologist working in neurorehabilitation. Claire has worked in diverse mental- and physical-health settings for over ten years, developing a passion for understanding the ways people can be supported to tell their life stories from a position of strength. She has a special interest in acquired brain injury, psychological resilience, and narrative therapy.

Part 1

Setting the Scene

1 Multicultural Neuropsychology

A UK Perspective

Ndidi Boakye

Introduction

Clinical neuropsychology is concerned with the relationship between brain dysfunction, cognition, emotion, and behaviour in everyday life. It is also tasked with the rehabilitation of individuals with cognitive, emotional, and behavioural problems arising from brain dysfunction. This is often achieved via neuropsychological assessment, where cognition, mood, and behaviour are all evaluated. The result of this assessment, often developed in collaboration with the multidisciplinary team, leads to an understanding of the consequences of brain injury on a patient's everyday functioning (Hart & Evans, 2006). Much of the work for the neuropsychologist and the neurorehabilitation team involves a combination of restoring and compensating for functional impairments and addressing the emotional consequences (Uomoto, 2015). Whilst this work is crucial, it can be circumscribed by a patient's cultural context. Much has been much written about the mismatch between patient goals and neurorehabilitation success (Van den Broek, 2005). In response, recommendations for a client-centred approach or value-based goal setting have followed to address this (Dekker et al., 2020). Despite these efforts, limited knowledge of the ways patients contribute to and navigate the social, historical, and political context they live in means that we as neuropsychologists risk missing vital opportunities to improve the quality of life for individuals with brain injury and their families/carers.

Health Outcomes for UK Ethnic Minorities

In recent years, the knowledge and awareness surrounding health inequalities have increased. The COVID-19 pandemic contributed much to this awareness raising. It took a greater toll on ethnic minority populations in the UK, stressing the role social determinants have in health and disease progression (Office for National Statistics, 2022). In this chapter, the terms *ethnic minorities* and *people of colour* will be used to refer to those socially racialised as non-White in the UK. We recognise that these terms are broad, reductionist, and Whiteness-centred. However, as these are the terms readily used in the literature that we draw from, we feel it is

DOI: 10.4324/9781003309819-2

necessary to use them, albeit cautiously, to capture neuropsychology in the current UK context. The term *Whiteness* will be used to refer to the systemic rules, norms, and discourses that produce and reproduce the dominance of those socially racialised as White. It is often invisible to its benefactors yet remains an oppressive reality to those socially racialised as people of colour (non-White ethnic groups). It is not synonymous with White people and can be reinforced by people of colour (DiAngelo, 2018).

In England, there is an increased recognition of health inequalities between ethnic minority and White groups, and between different ethnic minority groups. Studies have shown that rates of infant and maternal mortality, cardiovascular disease, and diabetes are higher among Black and South Asian groups (Raleigh & Holmes, 2021). Furthermore, prior to COVID, disability-free life expectancy was estimated to be lower among several ethnic minority groups compared with the White population. Raleigh and Holmes (2021) also highlight that people from ethnic minority groups are more likely to report being in poorer health and to report negative experiences of using health services than their White counterparts.

Researchers reported that ethnic minorities were at increased risk of medical conditions associated with cognitive impairments, such as stroke, epilepsy, myalgic encephalitis, and dementia (Hamdy et al., 2007; Bayliss et al., 2014; Pham et al., 2018). For example, Afro-Caribbeans and South Asians were twice as likely to suffer from a stroke (Department of Health, 2007). This is further compounded by higher rates of risk factors like diabetes and cardiovascular disease (Lievesley, 2010). Another study found that disease progression of multiple sclerosis is much quicker among Black Caribbean patients (Koffman et al., 2013).

There are multiple hypotheses about why these health disparities exist, including the increased risk being partially explained by situational factors, such as stressors in the role of a key worker and shift-work patterns (Franzen et al., 2021). There is another conversation to be had – a large body of research has established a causal relationship between experience of racial discrimination and adverse effects on mental and physical healthcare (Public Health England, 2020; Rao et al., 2020). Many racialised minority groups have described being targets of racism from law enforcement, health-care providers, educators, or employers, reminding us that racism occurs in all segments of our society. In this context, racial disparities – the phenomenon in which people of colour have poorer social and health outcomes than White people – are increasingly seen as evidence of systemic racism.

Access to Healthcare Services

Despite the increased risk of neurological conditions, individuals from minority backgrounds are underrepresented in neuropsychology services as both service users and staff members (Dunning & Teager, 2020;

Boakye et al., 2021). When compared to the 2011 census, White British individuals in referrals for outpatient and inpatient services were over-represented by 30%, whilst services users from an African background were underrepresented by 85%. South Asian service users were found to be underrepresented by 70%. This raises questions about how accessible neuropsychological services are for individuals from racialised minority backgrounds and how service user engagement can be increased.

Mirza et al. (2021) explored the potential factors that cause racial disparities within neuropsychology. It was identified that ethnic minority service users battled to access support, which triggered feelings of inequality and increased the distrust of medical professionals. The study found it was difficult for patients to understand their condition, as basic information on neurological conditions was not translated for non-English speakers (Mirza et al., 2021). Some of these factors are discussed further in Chapter 6 of this book.

Cognitive Assessments: Limitations and Barriers

The presentation of cognitive symptoms is an integral aspect of the assessment and diagnostic process for neurological conditions. Cognitive assessments involve a set of tasks that measure various skills, such as auditory and visual memory, language, and perceptual reasoning. Most neuropsychological assessments have been developed in English-speaking countries and standardised on individuals from English-speaking European and American backgrounds. Moreover, they cannot always be translated or culturally adapted (Franzen et al., 2021). We know already that neuropsychological test performance, administration, and results are impacted by numerous factors, such as culture, language, and ethnicity. In a cross-sectional qualitative and quantitative study, Baber (2020) identified a lack of neuropsychological instruments that account for cultural differences in the population. For instance, people from countries such as India, who have been educated in English, are subject to cross-cultural issues in test content despite not being at a linguistic disadvantage. In contrast, those who speak English as an additional language, like a White person who primarily speaks Welsh Cymraeg, can be disadvantaged linguistically on tests despite not encountering cross-cultural issues. Further research is required to understand the impact of cross-cultural and cross-linguistic differences and levels of acculturation in neurorehabilitation.

Fujii (2018) also stressed that experienced neuropsychologists may be well-versed in the standard process of conducting a neuropsychological evaluation, but they may still have difficulty determining a client's current functioning, given their unique cultural context. This is especially true when the service user and the clinician do not share the same ethnic background and language fluency. In such cases, the clinician risks administering a biased assessment with invalid tests, misinterpreted data, and inappropriate (if not harmful) treatment recommendations. Guidance on how to deliver culturally sensitive neuropsychological assessments is discussed in Chapter 6 and so will not be elaborated here. However, the question remains – how do we move from assessment to formulation, then on to safe treatment in neuropsychology when working cross-culturally?

Formulation in Neuropsychology

Klonoff, Stang, and Perumparaichallai (2017) state that it is the responsibility of the clinician to incorporate diversity factors in therapy. They rightly note that this mediates other psychological processes, such as the acceptance of disability, and supports reintegration back to one's social context. Formulation at its core is a provisional explanation or hypothesis of how an individual comes to present with a certain disorder or circumstance at a particular time (Weerasekera, 1996). It is also a tool that allows clinicians to relate theory to practise (Butler, 1998). The Division of Clinical Psychology (2011) defined it as a summation and integration of the knowledge that is acquired by the assessment process involving psychological, biological, systemic factors, and procedures.

The formulating clinician is required to be mindful of their positioning and the wider context within which the patient lives and the problem is constructed, such that the identified individual is not seen as the location of the problem (Johnstone & Dallos, 2013). In neuropsychology, formulation is guided by empirical and theoretical literature on cognitive functioning and utilises biopsychosocial and systemic models to develop an understanding of a patient's presentation (Wilson & Betteridge, 2019). Whilst this process is led by a clinical psychologist or neuropsychologist, input from the interdisciplinary team is crucial to ensure a holistic assessment and treatment. It is recommended that this process is conducted with the patient and/or their family and carers to develop a shared understanding of the problems and support engagement in rehabilitation (Wilson & Betteridge, 2019). Formulations are increasingly conducted at team level (Hollingworth & Johnstone, 2014), which allows clinical psychologists/neuropsychologists to demonstrate added value beyond individual interventions by using their consultation and leadership skills (Wood, 2016). Formulating psychologically with teams allows the identification of appropriate interventions, particularly for those with complex needs (Rainforth & Laurenson, 2014). The biopsychosocial model developed at the Oliver Zangwell Centre (Wilson et al., 2009a) has frequently been used to discuss complex cases. However, when working with ethnic minority groups there needs to be an appreciation of the multiple factors in the backdrop of people's lives.

David Smail (2005) describes the social environment as being the milieu which most substantially affects patients' lives. A social inequalities approach (McClelland, 2013) goes beyond the traditional boundaries of the biopsychosocial models, emphasising the role of social and cultural contexts in shaping problems. This is two-fold. Firstly, the structural features of society are seen as systematically marginalising and disempowering of some people and not others. Secondly, psychology itself is viewed as part of these structures, shaping how we think and feel about ourselves. Most important, this includes what we see as problematic behaviour. As multicultural neuropsychologists, we need to acknowledge that our work usually addresses the consequences of brain injury as well as broader-scale trauma on the local and personal level (microlevel) (Johnstone & Dallos, 2013) and on the intra-psychic or inter-personal level. However, the social inequalities perspective suggests that there are structural differences or hierarchies of power that limit and constrain some people and privilege others (Kagan et al., 2011). For example, if you are a working-age Black man with a stroke, it isn't enough to be referred to vocational rehabilitation. There has to be an acknowledgment that you faced barriers (racism and discrimination in obtaining and retaining employment) before. Therefore, now with a disability, you are less likely than your White counterpart to be employed. Knowledge of this by the psychologist will lead to the design of different interventions. There will be added awareness of the consequences for the individual and their social network of support.

If the formulation is fixed and little opportunity is offered to the patient to engage in the process, this may lead to disengagement from services. This may manifest earlier (or later) in the rehabilitation pathway – for example, when patients and families are making decisions about accepting care (on discharge or when referred to other services). Other decisions flowing from formulations include structured and prescriptive packages of care. When our patients do not ascribe to this, we describe them as not being 'ready for rehab' or not 'having goals'. This disconnect between professionals and patients leads to 'stuck' positions. Such processes are documented in the literature across a wide variety of psychological interventions (Del Re et al., 2012). Little thought is given to the psychological processes which may be driving these decisions for individuals and families, including shame, cultural values such as 'looking after your family', or the sense of 'not belonging'.

We propose the following model, which incorporates and then extends the Biopsychosocial model (Wilson et al., 2009b), to address this (Figure 1.1), and we use a case example to illustrate how taking an intersectionality perspective can shape the formulation and treatment outcomes.

Case Example

Hakeem was a 60-year-old Black man, who presented to the service with nocturnal epilepsy. He had been hit by a car at the age of 14, going head first into the windscreen. After being 'patched up', Hakeem was sent back to school. He complained of dizzy spells and headaches but

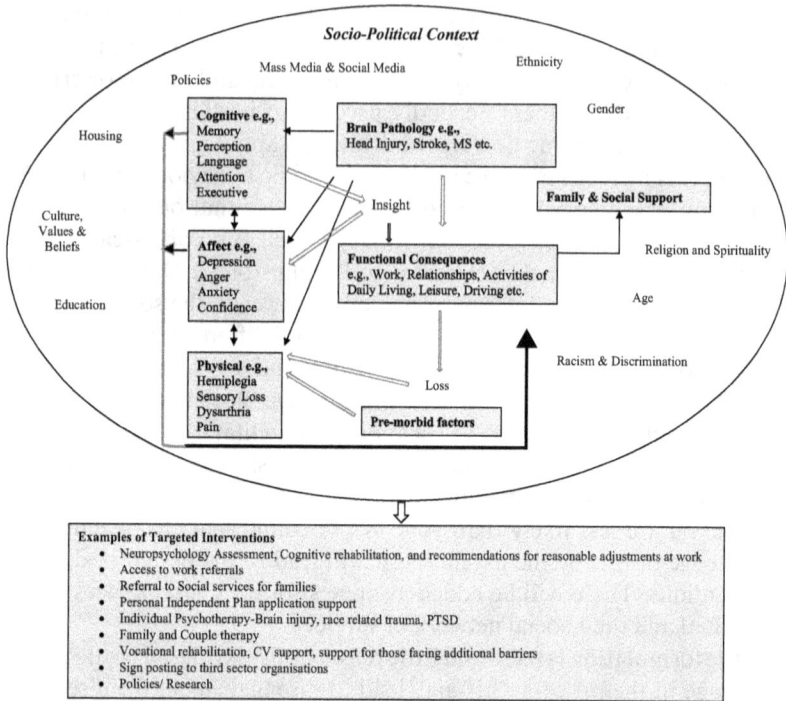

Figure 1.1 The Biopsychosocial Contextual Model of Brain Injury

was ignored by his teachers. His parents tried to seek support from the family GP, however his symptoms were dismissed as nothing serious. Hakeem was working towards A grades, but following the car accident he noticed it was harder to concentrate and remember information. He wanted to pursue carpentry as he was very creative and dexterous, however whilst in college one day, Hakeem had a fainting episode and could no longer pursue his course due to the safety risks involved. Hakeem changed his career trajectory and became a project manager despite resitting many exams due to ongoing memory difficulties. He went on to marry and have two children, but the dizziness persisted. These episodes increased in frequency over the years, and he was repeatedly dismissed over 11 visits to his GP. Hakeem did not receive adjustments at work, and he began to lose confidence in his abilities, leading to low mood. Following the death of his parents, Hakeem had a fall, and he pushed his GP for further investigations. An EEG and MRI scan confirmed a diagnosis of epilepsy secondary to a skull fracture relating to a previous brain injury. Therefore, he was eventually referred for a neuropsychology assessment of his reported memory difficulties at age 60.

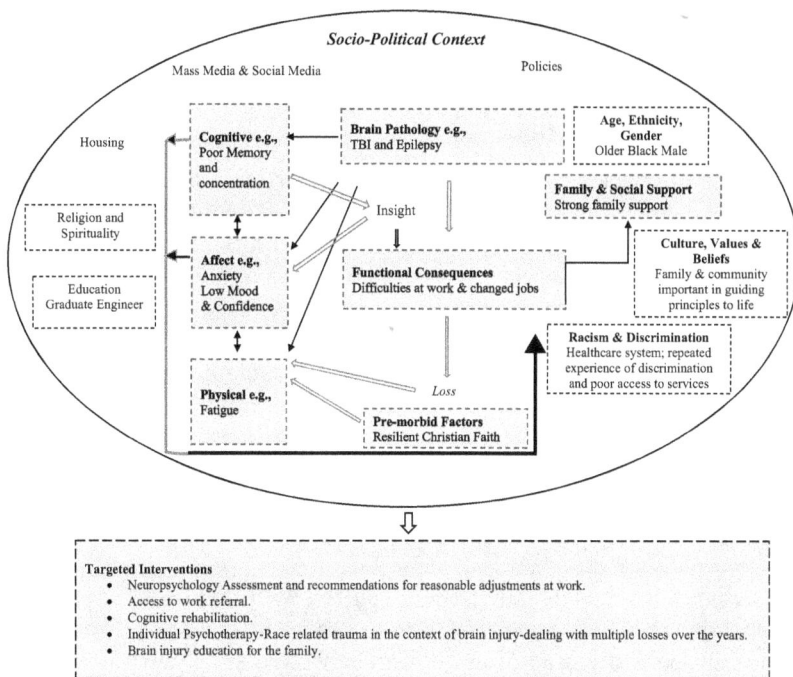

Figure 1.2 Hakeem's Formulation Model

Formulation

In the case study above, we see how structural barriers (e.g., lack of support from health services or the education system for Hakeem due to discrimination) meant that Hakeem was left with unaddressed cognitive complaints which impacted his social functioning, occupational trajectory, household income, and overall health outcome. The formulation model above (Figure 1.2) helps us to understand why he was not offered an assessment or rehabilitation straight after his initial brain injury. We know that there are significant differences in access to services across ethnic groups, so unsurprisingly there will be disparities in health outcomes, particularly physical health and psychological well-being (Kennedy, Kilvert, & Hasson, 2015). One might ask about the role of his parents; however, they would have likely faced the same barriers in trying to advocate for their son's well-being, coupled with years of psychological burnout from racism and discrimination. In Hakeem's case, treatment will not only involve neuropsychological assessment, but also further include family education on disability rights using the Equality Act (2010), reasonable adjustments available, Access to Work, eligibility for financial support via social service (personal independence plan), cognitive rehabilitation, psychotherapy for race-related trauma in the context of brain injury (loss of income, employment opportunities, identity), and couple and family therapy.

Treatment Considerations

The global prevalence of ABI is increasing, particularly in North America and Europe, where approximately 65 million people are affected every year (Dewan et al., 2018). Although community reintegration is the ultimate goal of rehabilitation post injury, ethnic minority populations continually face challenges with regards to unmet needs along the continuum of care, including meaningful participation and vocation, resulting in occupational deprivation (Omar, Nixon, & Colantanio, 2021). Baber (2020) highlighted that there is an underrepresentation of minoritised professionals in neuropsychology and limited training is available to educate neuropsychologists on how cultural variables affect treatment.

Neuropsychologists as Cultural Brokers

UK rehabilitation is usually patient-centred with the focus on personal independence, which is not the case in other cultures. For example, in some cultures illness and disability can be viewed as an inevitable aspect of ageing, so it is expected that the family will take on the burden of care rather than starting a rehabilitation programme (Hitchcock et al., 1998). Illness and disability can also be viewed from a spiritual or religious perspective, as discussed in Chapter 5. These cultural attitudes can also exist among patients within the UK (Barber, 2020). Studies have highlighted gaps at various stages of the service pathway from initial access to diagnosis to treatment, and further research is needed to examine facilitators and barriers to accessing neuropsychology services (Dunning & Teager, 2020; Boakye, Mobley, & Teager, 2021).

Perumparaichallai and Klonoff (2016) highlighted the different layers of culture in a milieu-oriented holistic neurorehabilitation program, including the culture of origin (e.g., Muslim), neurorehabilitation/milieu culture, brain injury culture, therapists' culture, and mainstream culture. In addition to this, healthcare providers are moulded by the culture of their profession (e.g., beliefs, practices/habits, norms, and rituals (Klonoff, Stang, & Perumparaichallai, 2017)). This often includes the use of medical terminology or jargon and setting of specific boundaries. This milieu creates a unique overall culture and means that the rehabilitation setting is not 'culture free' (Groce, 2005). How healthcare providers and patients navigate this unique environment when building a relationship is key. There are frequent meetings between staff and patients, with therapists holding knowledge about the neurological recovery process, compensatory strategies, and expectations. Sensitivity and awareness of the patient's cultural needs enables therapists to design treatment programs that are applicable to patients from ethnic minority groups (Perumparaichallai & Klonoff, 2016). Perumparaichallai and Klonoff (2016) suggest that the neuropsychologist can be useful in this context, acting as a cultural broker (bridging the gaps between groups or people of differing cultural backgrounds for the purpose of reducing conflict or producing change) by fostering a culturally sensitive and competent interdisciplinary team. Neuropsychologists can enable their teams to reflect on cultural considerations that arise in the clinical work. They also have a responsibility to be aware of their own positioning (e.g., gender, ethnicity, sexuality) and how that intersects with and impacts on their patients' positioning. Whilst previously there was an emphasis on cultural competency – 'the ability to engage knowledgeably with people across cultures' – which suggests an endpoint to becoming fully 'culturally competent'. Neuropsychologists are encouraged to move towards the newer framework of cultural humility and sensitivity, an idea discussed further in Chapter 11, which recognises the shifting nature of intersecting identities and encourages ongoing curiosity rather than an endpoint. Suggestions on how neuropsychologists can lead in a way that is sensitive to patients' social, cultural, and historical contexts are discussed.

Racial and Ethnic Microaggression

Uomoto (2016) suggests that there has been minimal discussion of the complex interpersonal dynamics that develop between cross-cultural dyads or recognition of its potential impact on the rehabilitation process. It is well documented in psychology and psychotherapy that one of the ways in which the working alliance or therapeutic relationship can be negatively impacted is when attitudes or prejudices are conveyed to patients and their families. This is usually in the form of racial and ethnic microaggression – that is, subtle (or not so subtle) insults (verbal, non-verbal, and/or visual) directed towards people of colour, often automatically or unconsciously. For example, a patient of colour attempts to discuss their feelings about being the only person of colour in the ward or experiencing alienation and dismissal by other patients, and the neuropsychologist replies, 'When I see you, I don't see colour' or 'I think you are being too paranoid, we should emphasise similarities, not people's differences'. Insensitivity by healthcare staff is unlikely to lead to positive treatment outcomes and reinforces experiences of racism and discrimination. Unfortunately, the power of microaggressions is in their subtle and ambiguous nature, which makes them hard to recognise and address (Hoffman, Rankin, & Loya, 2016). This also serves to keep them going. Cory (2021) concluded that White privilege in neuropsychology may in part explain some of the disparities seen in neuropsychological health outcomes. The insufficient systemic response to long-standing challenges related to workforce demographics and psychometric instruments was threatening neuropsychology's clinical relevance and utility. Cory (2021) stressed the need for neuropsychology to tackle the disconnect between an increasingly culturally and linguistically diverse population and the clinical tools currently available.

One way to do this might be to borrow from models in mental health – for example, the Assertive Outreach model. It is a way of organising and delivering care via a specialised team to provide intensive, highly coordinated but flexible support and treatment for individuals with longer-term needs living in the community. Community-based services could be modelled on this and offer more home-based rehabilitation packages. This could potentially increase engagement from minority groups in the community. So what is the way forward? Well, Baber (2020) has suggested that poor access to neuropsychological services as well as physical, political, and infrastructural barriers are linked to the underrepresentation of ethnic minority psychologists in neuropsychology. This underrepresentation is also likely to lead to poorer treatment (Baber, 2020). To move forward, neuropsychology must consider its workforce.

Neuropsychology and Workforce

In the 2021 May newsletter to the Division of Neuropsychology, Katherine Carpenter, the then chair of the Division of Neuropsychology, said,

> I was taken aback yet again to hear speakers, including Mivikeli Ncube and Nasreen Fazal-Short, speak about coming up against psychology views that Black and Brown people are less intelligent. Of course, I need to bear responsibility for poor science and racist psychology that has gone before. But I feel I need to go on record and say that neuropsychology today is certainly not based on or accepting of such views. Race is a social construct – a socio-political phenomenon not a biological one ... I put a heartfelt appeal out to all of you to help combat this misperception. After all, we all know perception is reality, so it's not enough that we know how things are, our Black and Brown patients and colleagues, the public, and everyone else also need to know how things are. So please have a think about what action you can take. Do we need to reassure patients before full assessment? Do we need to be explicit in our DClinPsy neuro modules, undergrad courses, and A-level teaching? What else can you do?
> (Division of Neuropsychology, 2021).

To answer Katherine, firstly, we (neuropsychologists) need to consider the pathway into Clinical Neuropsychology. To train and be recognised as a qualified clinical neuropsychologist in the UK, the criteria is that you must have the Health and Care Professions Council's (HCPC) registration as a Clinical, Educational, or Counselling Psychologist (QiCN, 2022). However, psychology as a discipline is under-representative of ethnic minorities, people with disabilities, and men, and it is increasingly skewed towards youth (Health Education England, 2021, p. 6). In order to increase diversity within the UK clinical neuropsychology workforce, we first need to tackle entry into applied psychology. This idea is discussed further in Chapter 13 of this book.

There is limited data on the ethnic backgrounds of psychologists and the impact of this on patient care. Furthermore, it has taken worldwide protests in June 2020 against the brutal murder of George Floyd; the COVID-19 pandemic health disparities; and the 2019 Group of Trainers in Clinical Psychology (GTiCP) conference, in which a re-enactment of a slave auction took place, for the British Psychological Society (BPS) to recognise racism within UK psychology (Bajwa, 2020). Discussion of racism in the profession has been a sensitive and often silenced issue (Howitt & Owusu-Bempah, 1994). Nonetheless, to move forward and ensure that we are providing a culturally sensitive and equitable service for all, clinical psychology – and therefore clinical neuropsychology – needs to take an active stance to address this issue. This includes the development of anti-racist practices, adopting a position of cultural humility, and ensuring that all psychologists are trained in attending to Whiteness, racism, and issues of culture in supervision, training, and practice (Wood & Patel, 2017).

Until these recommendations are adopted, Clinical Neuropsychology and other applied psychology professions will continue to deliver treatment and rehabilitation that potentially has an iatrogenic effect on some of its patients and their families. There is a need for planning and guidance, e.g., improving the curriculum, updating professional standards to include cultural competencies, and reflective practice on Whiteness, power, privilege, and intersectionality. In particular, neuropsychology needs to consider how to embed multicultural neuropsychology practices as a core part of the QiCN requirements. The world is changing fast, and we as neuropsychologists have the opportunity to further enhance our skills to deliver services that are culturally sensitive, high-standard, and equitable. Wars, and rumours of wars have increased immigration into the UK. There has never been a more important time to consider adapting and tailoring services to meet the diverse needs of a growing global UK population.

Conclusion

This chapter highlighted current limitations of clinical neuropsychology in an increasingly global UK context. It drew attention to the need to take into consideration the broader socio-political context when working with individuals and their families. Additionally, it proposed a new formulation model and offered case examples of how this work can be achieved. Challenges which can occur in the therapeutic relationship were discussed, such as racial microaggressions. Finally, it presented suggestions for how the professional can move forward, including improving the curriculum and updating professional standards to include cultural competencies and reflective practice on Whiteness, power, privilege, and intersectionality. This is an opportunity for neuropsychologists to further develop their clinical skills to deliver services that are sensitive, of the highest standard, and equitable.

References

Baber, Z. (2020). An exploration of the perspectives of neuropsychologists working with clients from ethnically, culturally and linguistically diverse backgrounds, Prof. Doc. Thesis, University of East London, School of Psychology.

Bajwa, S. (2020). Is the British Psychological Society institutionally racist? *The British Psychological Society.*

Bayliss, K., et al. (2014). Diagnosis and management of chronic fatigue syndrome/myalgic encephalitis in black and minority ethnic people: A qualitative study, *Prim Health Care Res Dev, 15*(2), 143–55.

Boakye, N., Mobley, A., & Teager, A. (2021, October 14–15). Evaluation of ethnicity in neuropsychology services. British Psychological Society Division of Neuropsychology Conference 2021.

Butler, P. V. (1998). Psychology as history, and the biological renaissance: A brief review of the science and politics of psychological determinism, *Australian Psychologist, 33*, 40–46.

Cory, J. J. (2021). White privilege in neuropsychology: An 'invisible knapsack' in need of unpacking?, *The Clinical Neuropsychologist, 35*(2), 206–18.

Dekker, J., de Groot, V., Ter Steeg, A. M., Vloothuis, J., Holla, J., Collette, E., ... & Littooij, E. (2020). Setting meaningful goals in rehabilitation: Rationale and practical tool, *Clinical Rehabilitation, 34*(1), 3–12.

Del Re, A. C., Flückiger, C., Horvath, A. O., Symonds, D., & Wampold, B. E. (2012). Therapist effects in the therapeutic alliance-outcome relationship: A restricted-maximum likelihood meta-analysis, *Clinical Psychology Review, 32*(7), 642–49.

Department of Health. (2007). *Department of Health National Stroke Strategy.*

Dewan, M. C., Rattani, A., Gupta, S., Baticulon, R. E., Hung, Y. C., Punchak, M., ... & Park, K. B. (2018). Estimating the global incidence of traumatic brain injury, *Journal of Neurosurgery, 130*(4), 1080–97.

DiAngelo, R. (2018). *White fragility: Why it's so hard for white people to talk about racism.* Beacon Press.

Division of Clinical Psychology. (2011). *Good practice guidelines on the use of psychological formulation.* British Psychological Society.

Division of Neuropsychology (2021, May) Division of Neuropsychology Conference, *British Psychological Society.*

Dunning, G., & Teager, A. (2020, November). An evaluation of ethnicity in a neuropsychology outpatient department. Division of Clinical Psychology Annual Conference. https://www.researchgate.net/publication/343255580_An_evaluation_of_ethnicity_in_a_neuropsychology_outpatient_department.

Franzen, S., Papma, M., Berg, E., & Nielsen, T. (2021). Cross-cultural neuropsychological assessment in the European Union: A Delphi expert study, *Archives of Clinical Neuropsychology, 36*(5), 815–30.

Fujii, D. E. (2018). Developing a cultural context for conducting a neuropsychological evaluation with a culturally diverse client: The ECLECTIC framework.
The Clinical Neuropsychologist, 32(8), 1356–92.

Groce, N. (2005). Immigrants, disability, and rehabilitation. In J. H. Stone
(Ed.), *Culture and disability: Providing culturally competent services* (pp. 1–14).
SAGE.

Hamdy, N. A., et al. (2007). Ethnic differences in the incidence of seizure disorders in children from Bradford, United Kingdom. *Epilepsia, 48*(5), 913–16.

Hart, T., & Evans, J. (2006). Self-regulation and goal theories in brain injury
rehabilitation. *The Journal of Head Trauma Rehabilitation, 21*(2), 142–55.

Health Education England. (2021). *Psychological Professionals Workforce Plan for
England: The Psychological Professions Professional groups in the NHS in En-
gland.* https://www.hee.nhs.uk/sites/default/files/documents/Psychological%20
Professions%20Workforce%20Plan%20for%20England%20-%20Final.pdf.

Hitchcock, R., Hutchings, C. J., Stephenson, S., & Ward, C. D. (1998). Neurological rehabilitation in Indonesia and the UK: Differences and similarities.
Journal of Allied Health, 27(1), 45–49.

Hoffman, J., Rankin, R., & Loya, K. (2016). Climate as a Mediating Influence
on the Perceived Academic Success of Women Student-Athletes, *Journal
for the Study of Sports and Athletes in Education, 10*(3), 164–84. DOI:
10.1080/19357397.2016.1256047.

Hollingworth, P., & Johnstone, L. (2014). Team formulation: What are the staff
views. *Clinical Psychology Forum, 257*(5), 28–34.

Howitt, D., & Owusu-Bempah, J. (1994). *The Racism of Psychology: Time for
Change.* Harvester Wheatsheaf.

Johnstone, L., & Dallos, R. (2013). Introduction to formulation. In L. Johnstone &
R. Dallos (Eds.), *Formulation in psychology and psychotherapy* (pp. 21–37).
Routledge.

Kagan, C., Burton, M., Duckett, P., Lawthom, R., & Siddiquee, A. (2011). *Critical Community Psychology* (1st ed.). Wiley-Blackwell.

Kennedy P., Kilvert, A., & Hasson, L. (2015). Ethnicity and Rehabilitation
Outcomes: The Needs Assessment Checklist. *Spinal Cord, 53*(5), 334–39. DOI:
10.1038/sc.2015.14.

Klonoff, P. S., Stang, B., & Perumparaichallai, K. (2017). Family-Based
Support for People with Brain Injury. In B. A. Wilson, J. Winegardner, C.
M van Heugten, & T. Ownsworth, *Neuropsychological Rehabilitation: The
International Handbook* (pp. 364–77). Routledge.

Koffman, J., Gao, W., Goddard, C., Burman, R., Jackson, D., … & Higginson,
I.J. (2013) Progression, Symptoms and Psychosocial Concerns among Those
Severely Affected by Multiple Sclerosis: A Mixed-Methods Cross-Sectional
Study of Black Caribbean and White British People. *PLoS ONE, 8*(10): e75431.
DOI:10.1371/journal.pone.0075431.

Lievesley, N. (2010). *The future ageing of the ethnic minority population of England
and Wales.* Runnymede.

McClelland, L. (2013). Reformulating the impact of social inequalities. In L.
Johnstone & R. Dallos (Eds.), *Formulation in psychology and psychotherapy:
Making sense of people's problems* (pp. 121–44). Routledge.

Mirza, N., Vikram, A., Osmani, F., Kumar, N., Orakzai, S., Sharma, S., & Ehsan,
S. (2021). *Barriers and facilitators British ethnic minorities face when accessing*

neuropsychological services: A systematic review and qualitative analysis. British Psychological Society Conference. DOI: 10.13140/RG.2.2.21383.32167.

Office for National Statistics. (2022). Updating ethnic contrasts in deaths involving the coronavirus (COVID-19), England, 8 December 2020 to 1 December 2021. https://www.ons.gov.uk/peoplepopulationandcommunity/birthsdeathsandmarriages/deaths/articles/updatingethniccontrastsindeathsinvolvingthecoronaviruscovid19englandandwales/8december2020to1december2021.

Omar, S., Nixon, S., & Colantonio, A. (2021). Integrated Care Pathways for Black Persons With Traumatic Brain Injury: A Critical Transdisciplinary Scoping Review of the Clinical Care Journey. *Trauma, Violence, & Abuse*, DOI: 10.1177%2F15248380211062221.

Perumparaichallai, K., & Klonoff, P. (2016). Layers of Culture: Its influence in a milieu-oriented holistic neurorehabilitation setting, In J. M. Uomoto (Ed.), *Multicultural Neurorehabilitation: Clinical Principles for Rehabilitation Professionals* (pp. 119–38). Springer.

Pham, T. M., et al. (2018). Trends in dementia diagnosis rates in UK ethnic groups: Analysis of UK primary care data. *Clinical Epidemiology, 10*, 949–60.

Public Health England. (2020). *Disparities in the risk and outcomes of COVID-19.* PHE Publications.

QiCN (Qualification in Clinical Neuropsychology). (2022). *QiCN 2022 Handbook for Candidates.* British Psychological Society.

Rainforth, M., & Laurenson, M. (2014). A literature review of case formulation to inform mental health practice. *Journal of Psychiatric and Mental Health Nursing, 21*(3), 206–13.

Raleigh, V., & Holmes, J. (2021, September 17). The health of people from ethnic minority groups in England. *The King's Fund.* https://www.kingsfund.org.uk/publications/health-people-ethnic-minority-groups-england.

Rao, A., Hemmingfield, J., & Greenhill, B. (2020). *Racial and Social Inequalities: Taking the conversation forward. DCP Racial and Social Inequalities in the Times of Covid-19 Working Group.* British Psychological Society.

Smail, D. J. (2005). *Power, interest and psychology: Elements of a social materialist understanding of distress.* PCCS Books.

Uomoto, J. M. (2015). *Multicultural neurorehabilitation: Clinical principles for rehabilitation professionals.* Springer Publishing Company.

Uomoto, J. M. (2016). The contribution of the neuropsychological evaluation to traumatic brain injury rehabilitation. In M. J. Ashley & D. A. Hovda (Eds.), *Traumatic Brain Injury: Rehabilitation, Treatment and Case Management* (pp. 859–98). CRC Press.

Van den Broek, M. D. (2005). Why does neurorehabilitation fail? *Journal of Head Trauma Rehabilitation, 20*(5), 464–73.

Weerasekera, P. (1996). *Multi perspective case formulation: A step towards treatment integration.* Krieger Publishing Company.

Wilson, B. A., & Betteridge, S. (2019). *Essentials of neuropsychological rehabilitation.* Guilford Publications.

Wilson, B. A., Gracey, F., Evans, J. J., & Bateman, A. (2009a). *Neuropsychological rehabilitation: Theory, models, therapy and outcome.* Cambridge University Press.

Wilson, B. A., Gracey, F., Malley, D., Bateman, A., & Evans, J. (2009b). The Oliver Zangwill centre approach to neuropsychological rehabilitation. In B.

A. Wilson, F. Gracey, J. J. Evans, & A. Bateman (Eds.), *Neuropsychological rehabilitation: Theory, models, therapy and outcome* (pp. 47–67). Cambridge University Press

Wood, K. (2016). *Clinical Psychologists' Experiences of Moving Towards Using Team Formulation in Multidisciplinary Settings.* University of Surrey (United Kingdom).

Wood, N., & Patel, N. (2017). On addressing 'Whiteness' during clinical psychology training. *South African Journal of Psychology, 47*(3), 280–29.

Part 2

Diversity Matters in System Working

2 Good Teams Mind Their GGRRAAACCCEEESSS

Ndidi Boakye, Amanda Mwale and Camille Julien

Introduction

Patients in healthcare present with a number of complexities, from their physical health condition to the additional layer of accompanying psychological sequelae. In order to meet their needs, clinicians need to work together to develop a shared understanding. It is recommended that patients are discussed and treated by a team of dedicated specialists (Department of Health, 2005) to ensure that they receive the best possible care. This is known as a multi-disciplinary team (MDT). The team works together to create a treatment plan and do so by developing a shared understanding of the difficulties presented. This shared understanding promotes person-centred care by summarising the psychological, biological, and systemic factors that cause and maintain a person's condition (Division of Clinical Psychology, 2011).

Team Formulation

Team formulation has been described as a process of facilitating a group of professionals to construct a shared understanding of a service user's difficulties (Johnstone & Dallos, 2013). Psychologists are key in this process as they are trained to draw on theories and models to develop an understanding of a person's experiences, difficulties, strengths, and resources. Hypotheses are subsequently generated with the aim to develop an explanation that facilitates both decision-making and interventions underpinned by psychological theory. Working psychologically with teams is considered a way for clinical psychologists to utilise skills such as formulation to support other clinicians in identifying an appropriate intervention, particularly for those with complex needs (Rainforth & Laurenson, 2014).

Team formulation can provide a safe space for staff to express feelings evoked by working with people with complex health conditions and psychological difficulties. They allow for these feelings to be contained and 'detoxified' (Holmes, 2002; Summers, 2006). It may also minimise 'splitting' within teams, improve team cohesion, reduce work-related stress, and minimise burnout (Kerr, Dent-Brown, & Parry, 2007).

DOI: 10.4324/9781003309819-4

Furthermore, team formulation can increase staff knowledge, develop shared care, increase multidisciplinary working, improve dissemination of information (Craven-Staines, Dexter-Smith, & Li, 2010), guide systemic changes to care (Taylor & Sambrook, 2012; Moore & Drennan, 2013), and provide meaning and direction to nursing care (Crowe, Carlyle, & Farmar, 2008). Thus, the goals of team formulation are to improve staff knowledge and skills and to improve care experiences and outcomes (Holmes, 2002; Kerr, Dent-Brown, & Parry, 2007). The use of team formulation to support MDT members has had a positive impact on care planning, staff-patient relationships, and staff satisfaction, increasing understanding of patients, team working, and intervention planning and promoting psychological mindedness (Craven-Staines, Dexter-Smith, & Li, 2010; Hollingworth & Johnstone, 2014; Wainwright & Bergin, 2010).

The benefits of team formulation have been recognised by both clinical psychologists and non-psychologist staff members (Christofides, Johnstone, & Musa, 2012; Hood, Johnstone, & Christofides, 2013). Berry, Barrowclough, and Wearden (2009) investigated the effects of team formulation informed by a Cognitive Interpersonal Model in an inpatient psychiatric rehabilitation setting. Half of the wards were randomised to staff use of formulation plus treatment as usual (TAU) or TAU only. Compared to TAU, service users who received care from staff using team formulation felt less criticised by staff and also reported less emotional distance from staff. In a study focussing on older people, Murphy, Osborne, and Smith (2013) used thematic analysis to explore the views of nurses regarding psychological formulation, using a team approach, within an older people's mental health inpatient service. The formulation approach was based on a model developed by Dexter-Smith (2007). A three-day training package for staff regarding the approach was followed by weekly formulation sessions with staff led by a Clinical Psychologist. The findings were consistent with those of other team formulation studies, suggesting that the approach increases staff understanding of patients, helps staff tolerate difficult feelings, and improves team working (Summers, 2006; Berry, Barrowclough, & Wearden, 2009). The findings further suggested that team formulation can lead to modification of care for patients and enable teams to develop a unified and consistent approach to care.

Team Formulation in Neurorehabilitation

Despite the positives highlighted above, there is limited research conducted on how to implement team formulation (Wood, 2016), and research has identified inconsistencies in the way that team formulation is utilised in services (Cole, Wood, & Spendelow, 2015). There is a gap in research for the use of team formulation within neurorehabilitation services. Wilson and Betteridge (2019) recommend a holistic biopsychosocial formulation approach in neurorehabilitation teams that places the patient at the centre and incorporates all aspects of the system surrounding the individual to help identify rehabilitation needs. Whilst a clinical psychologist/neuropsychologist may lead this process, they suggest that interdisciplinary working will help promote a holistic assessment that provides a thorough understanding of the individual. However, they caution that this process is conducted transparently with the patient and/or their family and carers. This promotes a shared understanding of the problems and can facilitate motivation to engage in the rehabilitation programme (Wilson & Betteridge, 2019). These meetings can occur monthly, and the focus is to discuss one complex case with a view to developing a shared formulation that will guide intervention planning. This approach is aimed at promoting joint working, the use of shared team formulation, and goal setting in line with models of best practice in neurorehabilitation settings (Wilson & Betteridge, 2019). However, more research is needed to assess the value in integrating neuropsychological formulation within clinical practice.

The Social GGRRAAACCEEESSS and Team Formulation

The Social GGRRAAACCEEESSS framework developed by Burnham (1992) and Roper-Hall (1998) is increasingly used as a framework across clinical and education settings to encourage the critical exploration of social differences (Birdsey & Kustner, 2020). They have been extended in recent years from the initial nine to 15 areas to include: Gender, Geography, Race, Religion, Age, Ability, Appearance, Class, Culture, Ethnicity, Education, Employment, Sexuality, Sexual orientation and Spirituality (Burnham, 2018). The aim is to enable clinicians and or learners to become more alert to any biases that may impact on the therapeutic or treatment process. Each element of the GGRRAAACCEEESSS is equally important (Nolte, 2017); however, anecdotal evidence suggests clinicians have a propensity to explore issues that they privilege or feel most skilled in focusing on (Burnham, Palma, & Whitehouse, 2008). Supervision therefore becomes instrumental in orienting clinicians to consider aspects of the patient's (and their families') lived experience that have not been attended to, thereby promoting an understanding of the impact of socio-political context on families. The use of this framework in team formulation approaches is therefore crucial. However, although social GGRRAAACCEEESSS can help clinicians attend to (un)voiced or (in)visible differences and the varying aspects of power that follow, it can oversimplify the uniqueness and complexities of the privileges and oppressions created at intersections of clinicians and patients' social locations (Butler, 2015). The concept of intersectionality, which denotes how one is simultaneously positioned – for example, as Black, disabled, working-class, lesbian, or colonial subject (Crenshaw, 1991) – bridges this gap by allowing the 'both/and' position (Burnham, 1999). When leading team formulations, it is important that psychologists facilitate other members of the MDT to hold in mind the concept of intersectionality during case discussions in order for clinicians to understand the lived experience of their patients.

In their recent systematic review of team formulation, Geach, Moghaddam, and De Boos (2018) identified three instantiations of team formulation: sharing ideas informally, reflective practice meetings, and formulation-focussed consultation. In the examples below, we discuss how we have used the different instantiation of team formulation approaches in our clinical work.

Reflective Practice: The Reflecting Team Model

The reflecting team model can be used by groups of clinician. Training is not required to participate; however, instructions on how to use the space can be helpful in facilitating participation (see Box 2.1). Ground rules are established, such as confidentiality, respect for the opinions of others, and allowing each person to talk.

Box 2.1

Ways of offering reflections:

- Positively reframe what has been said,
- Reflect on different understandings,
- Use personal experience or previous cases,
- Ask hypothetical questions, or
- Say how we have been affected by what we've heard.

The psychologist takes the role of an interviewer/facilitator and 'interviews' a person (case presenter) or a small team that brings a clinical or professional dilemma to the group. Details of the case are clarified with the case presenter, after which the facilitator asks the case presenter what questions or support they would like from the group. The case presenter and the facilitator then face away from the group and avoid any direct eye contact – for example, by turning their chairs away or sitting a few metres away. The group proceeds to discuss the case using the questions raised by the case presenter. The hope is that new perspectives open up for the case presenter. When used in neurorehabilitation settings, teams report 'enjoying' the process and 'being surprised' at the new perspectives that come up.

For example, one neurorehabilitation team presented a 'safeguarding' concern at a reflective practice session. In this case example, members of the MDT were on a home visit with a 56-year-old woman who had had a stroke. This woman lived at home with her 21-year-old daughter and 18-year-old son. The son was typically absent, but the daughter was always home to let the physiotherapist and occupational therapist into the home. The team members were very concerned because the front of the house was unruly, the rose bushes were overgrown, and the ambulance crew had such difficulty wheeling the patient out of the house that they now refused to collect her for weekly sessions. The team therefore decided to provide her rehabilitation at home; however, they were finding it challenging as the home was unkempt and there were food packages left in bedrooms. The team reported discussing this with the daughter but felt that she was quite dismissive. They wondered if the mother was being neglected, but when they raised this with her, she defended her children, reporting that they did their best and, although not immediately responsive, did eventually get round to tidying things up.

With support from the psychologist, the reflective team opened the conversation up and they considered the GGRRAAACCEEESSS that had not been attended to. This included discussing the ethnicity of the family. Questions were asked about engagement with services, including reflections about previous 'relationship to help' (Reder & Fredman, 1996) and the challenge for a Black family living with disability to accept support from an all-White team. New information came to light, such as the fact that the daughter was pregnant, and the team questioned if this may be why it was difficult for her to be expected to tidy the house and raised concerns about her well-being and if this was or had been addressed? The team were also curious about the role of the son. How involved was he? What expectations did the team have about his involvement in care for his mother, and did his age, gender, and life stage impact expectations? Did we as a health team have different expectations for them as a Black family? These conversations enabled the case presenter to take on a more compassionate stance towards the family and, rather than considering solely a safeguarding approach, to recognise that perhaps this was a family that required further tailored support from services.

In our clinical experiences, teams have often reported reflective spaces as refreshing and useful in generating multiple hypotheses for their patients. The next section is a case example offered by one of the authors (CJ) about their experience of offering a reflective space for their team.

Good Teams Mind Their GGRRAAACCEEESSS

I (CJ) had just started working as a clinical psychologist on the stroke pathway in a busy, metropolitan hospital that covered a large and diverse population characterised by stark socioeconomic and health inequalities. The multidisciplinary teams (MDTs) along the pathway (acute and early supported discharge teams) were well established, highly skilled, and compassionate towards their patients and their families. However, they faced high levels of stress and burnout due to the demands of working with a large caseload of patients with high levels of socioeconomic deprivation, complex psychosocial backgrounds, and comorbid physical and mental health challenges.

Furthermore, chronic staff shortages in the Trust meant staff had to stretch their resources in order to meet clinical demands. Staff reported a lack of confidence in their ability to manage the psychological impacts of brain injury on stroke survivors and their families. I noticed that certain short-hand terms were commonly used to describe the behaviour of individuals whom the team had difficulty engaging (e.g., 'behavioural', 'unmotivated', 'noncompliant', 'obstructive'), with little time taken to understand what other factors beyond brain injury or personality might contribute to making interactions challenging for staff. This seemed particularly pertinent as the therapy staff were mostly White, middle-class, British women between the ages of 25 and 45 working with patients and families from very different socioeconomic, ethnic, cultural, and religious backgrounds and with a wide range of ages.

I reflected on the role a psychologist might play in supporting the team to deliver person-centred, holistic care and the need to develop an accessible framework that would enable staff to look beyond the surface of an interaction and consider the layers of personal, family, and cultural meaning that might influence how care and rehabilitation is understood and negotiated in healthcare settings. This approach fitted well with the recommended matched care model of psychological care in stroke, where the MDT is trained and supported to provide basic psychological care to stroke survivors and their families (Bowen, James, & Young, 2016). It also allowed me to draw on my systemic training and, in particular, models such as Pearce and Cronen's (1980) Coordinated Management of Meaning, a social-constructionist theory that posits that individuals construct their own social realities through interactions with others, and social realities are heavily influenced by one's personal and socio-cultural context, so that communication is at greater risk of breaking down when individuals operate from different contexts.

I developed a one-day training for the whole MDT entitled 'Level 1 training in psychological care' that covered understanding the psychological needs of stroke survivors and their families, the management of difficult conversations in limited time, concerns to look out for and referring on, and self-care and supporting each other (Julien & Simkiss, 2013). A core part of the training was developing skills in formulating challenging healthcare situations from a holistic, systemic perspective. I used the widely used metaphor of the iceberg to guide the team in their reflection (see Figure 2.1).

In this framework, the iceberg represents the patient/family member that the staff member is interacting with, the ship represents the staff

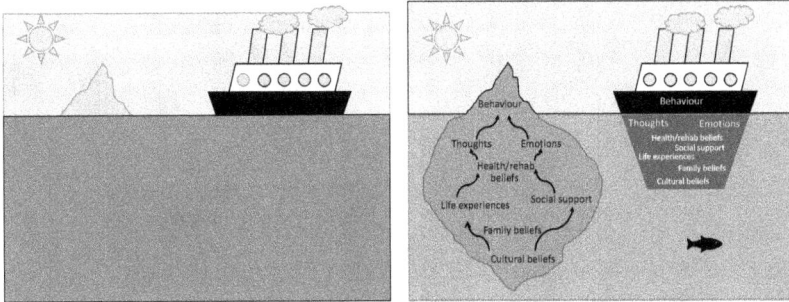

Figure 2.1 Iceberg Metaphor to Guide Teams in Reflections

member, and the sea represents the specific healthcare setting (e.g., inpatient unit, community). Both the iceberg and the ship have a visible part, which represents overt behaviour/speech, and a hidden part under the surface, which represents the beliefs, life experiences, family, and social and cultural values that may be driving the visible behaviour. Although interactions are often harmonious, clashes, misunderstandings, and disengagement may occur (i.e., the ship and iceberg collide) when there is a mismatch below the surface between 'hidden' personal, social, and cultural narratives. During the training workshop, staff were invited to think of a case from their professional experience and use the iceberg framework to formulate the factors relating both to the patient and themselves that may have contributed to a challenging interaction. The strength of this framework is that it incorporates not only a holistic formulation of the patient but also allows the staff member to consider their own context and how this influences their interactions at work. The framework can be applied to any situation, whether it be a conversation with a stroke survivor, their family member, or even another colleague. Following the one-day training workshop, staff were asked to complete a case reflection using the iceberg model and share it with the group at a half-day follow-up workshop six weeks later. Monthly case reflections were then put in place for the MDT to continue to build their reflective skills and develop cohesive, coordinated plans for person-centred care, and the iceberg framework was used as a way of making sense of the team's experiences whilst engaging with specific clinical scenarios.

Figure 2.2 demonstrates an example of a case that was brought to the follow-up workshop. A young, White, British, female physiotherapist in the Early Supported Discharge team had been working with a Bangladeshi, Muslim stroke survivor in his 60s. Although she felt he had good potential to make a physical recovery, she was increasingly frustrated by his seeming lack of engagement in rehabilitation and reluctance to leave the house and try activities that she felt would help increase his

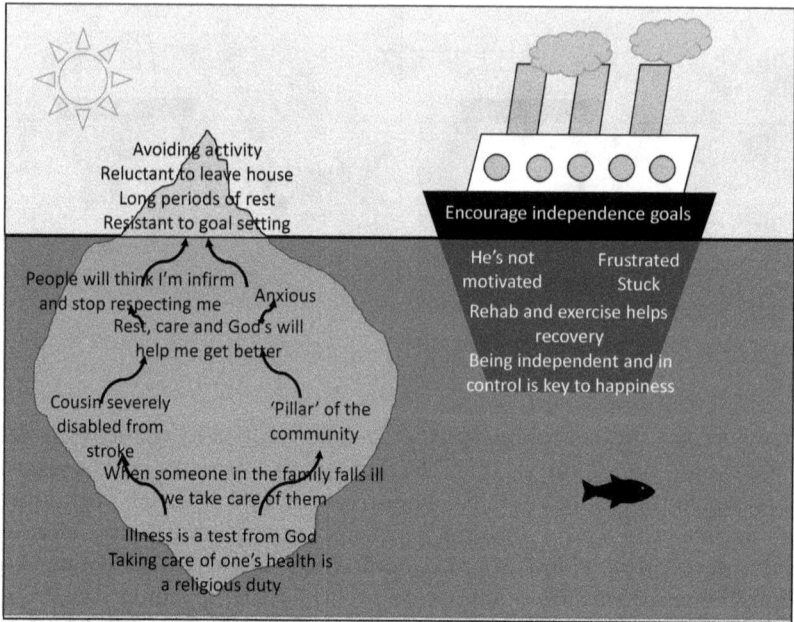

Avoiding activity
Reluctant to leave house
Long periods of rest
Resistant to goal setting

Encourage independence goals

People will think I'm infirm
and stop respecting me   Anxious
Rest, care and God's will
help me get better

He's not   Frustrated
motivated   Stuck
Rehab and exercise helps
recovery
Being independent and in
control is key to happiness

Cousin severely   'Pillar' of the
disabled from   community
stroke
When someone in the family falls ill
we take care of them

Illness is a test from God
Taking care of one's health is
a religious duty

Figure 2.2 An Example of the Iceberg Metaphor Applied to a Clinical Scenario

independence. Any discussion about goals would lead to resistance on his part, and she was considering discharging him, as she felt he was 'not motivated' to make progress.

The iceberg model reflection led her to develop professional curiosity about his context. He was able to share his belief that rest and care would aid his recovery and his belief in 'God's will'. He also shared his anxiety about being seen by others as 'infirm' and, as a result, losing his standing in the community. She was able to reflect on her own implicit beliefs about the primacy of independence and autonomy, influenced by her Western culture, and her strong beliefs about the importance of rehabilitation and exercise in stroke recovery. Coming from an atheist family, she had not considered the relevance of religious faith to recovery. Gaining this understanding helped her negotiate physical goals that were more connected to his religious values (e.g., walking to the mosque, kneeling for prayer) while respecting his need for rest and care. She was also able to include his family in the rehabilitation plan, and she referred to the psychologist to support him in managing his worries about social identity and adjusting to living as a stroke survivor in his community. The role of the psychologist here cannot be underestimated. By enabling the physiotherapist to be curious about her own biases, the trajectory of this patient's journey was changed. Nonetheless, it is important to acknowledge that it can be challenging for clinicians to find time in a busy rehabilitation setting to attend reflective team meetings. However, there are other forums in which these spaces can be created.

Supporting 'Minding our GGRRAAACCEEESSS' in Multidisciplinary Meetings

In a fast-paced neurorehabilitation setting, the MDT meeting can be an ideal environment for sharing formulations as well as supporting teams to reflect on the impact of a variety of GGRRAAACCEEESSS at play in their work.

Case Example

It's 8:45 a.m., and the multidisciplinary team have commenced their weekly meeting to discuss the progress of medical and therapy interventions for a number of patients accessing intensive Level 1 neurorehabilitation. They have started to discuss 'Ade', a 43-year-old patient of Nigerian descent. He was admitted to the hospital after experiencing a stroke, which has affected his speech, cognitive skills, and mobility. He has been on the ward for ten days. His lead clinician, a White, British, female occupational therapist in her 30s, says, 'I don't think he's suitable for rehab here. He is not engaging, and he is now getting aggressive. It's getting unsafe to approach him'.

The incident of aggression was reportedly a situation where the gentleman attempted to hit a therapist with a walking aid. A few other members of the team, which includes a speech and language therapist, nurse, and physiotherapist, contribute and share stories about his disengagement and refusal to be supported when showering or to attend therapy sessions. Subsequently, the psychologist present asks the team what is known about the patient's background context. The lead clinician goes on to share that, prior to the stroke, Ade had been living in an unkempt room in a shared flat and worked as a part-time caretaker. On inspection of his rented bedroom, an old photograph of a woman and child was found as well as a rolled up degree certificate in Business Studies obtained at a university in Nigeria. The gentleman had no known social contacts apart from the woman who was subletting the flat he was living in. She shared that he was studying for a course at the local college and knew him to be a 'loner'.

In the example above, the psychologist drew attention to the patient's social circumstances in order to prompt the team to slow down and focus on the broader picture of Ade's situation. The details highlighted above then prompted further questions and challenged the team to attend to the needs of the patient that the team were unable to access when their agenda (meeting MDT-set goals) was their priority. The team was subsequently asked further questions, including: Do we know who the individuals in the photograph are? Is he is missing or worried about somebody whilst being in hospital? How long has he lived in the UK? How must he feel because his current work is misaligned with his education? What threats do the neurorehabilitation setting present for him? All of these questions led to a more comprehensive and compassionate formulation of Ade's situation. It allowed for a better understanding of his behaviours, which seemed to communicate his desire to remain in control in confusing, unexpected, and distressing circumstances. This led therapists to make changes to the way they approached Ade, such as offering clearer explanations about what they were about to do, asking him questions, offering more choices, and giving him more time to make his own decisions with support.

A further exploration involved investigating the 'aggressive incident', including what may have triggered it and how it unfolded. Discussions with the staff members involved revealed that Ade had been startled when approached and lost his balance, which led to his walking stick being flicked upwards. The incident was misinterpreted, which led to an unhelpful narrative about his behaviour and intentions – to hurt those who wanted to help him – which was not the case. In addition, upon further reflection on this work, reflective practice for the team also would have been a very useful learning opportunity about the impact of microaggressions. Racial microaggressions are defined as subtle verbal or non-verbal behaviours, racial slights, or insults that are demeaning, hostile, or disrespectful towards people of colour, and they may be intentional or unintentional (Sue et al., 2007). It was important for the team to be reminded of how easy it is for microaggressions against Black patients to occur due to implicit biases and racial stereotypes people held as well as of the impact this could have in practice.

Looking After Our Nurses: Responding to Inequalities and Discrimination

Our experiences have demonstrated that it is vital to attend to inequalities and experiences of discrimination against members of staff with protected characteristics, which includes race. It is well documented that a large proportion of ethnic minority nurses report experiences of racist behaviour from colleagues and patients (e.g., Likupe, 2006). In addition, therapists and medical teams are often at the centre of decision-making relating to patient neurorehabilitation, and nursing staff are often required to implement plans rather than influence them. This means that nurses also often hold unequal power in relation to other professions within neurorehabilitation and can feel undervalued (Miller & Kontos, 2013). Therefore, ethnic minority nurses can experience disadvantage from discrimination against their racial identity as well as their professional identity. An example includes our experiences working with nursing staff who have experienced racial microaggressions and abuse from patients with challenging behaviours as well as from colleagues who may exclude nurses from contributing to plans to manage these behaviours. Due to having had a brain injury, patients' racist comments and actions can sometimes be dismissed as 'behavioural' and 'impulsive' by other colleagues and the recipients themselves. As a result, the emotional impact of these hurtful discriminative experiences goes unaddressed and adds to the cumulative stress that staff from minoritised backgrounds might experience in the workplace. Sometimes these experiences may also be vicarious (distress arising from being a witness to discrimination and aggression). It is important that staff support is timely and responsive following these experiences. These issues are discussed further in Chapter 8.

A vital role for supervising or supporting clinicians is to ensure that staff are offered a safe space to discuss their experiences of discrimination and aggression. Therefore, both group and/or individual support sessions should be offered as options. In our experience, nursing staff have demonstrated very varied responses to racist behaviour in both individual and group support sessions. Some nursing staff have been vocal and expressed their anger, some remained silent and suppressed their experiences, whilst others have presented with intense distress.

A range of various understandable feelings can emerge, such as anger, anxiety, powerlessness, shame, and hurt. A helpful support session requires the listener to be sensitive to the needs of the staff member(s) and to listen without judgement, thus avoiding invalidation of their distress. Staff sharing their experiences should also be assured that action will take place to support them further and to minimise their exposure to future incidents where possible. For example, one of the actions may include formulating behavioural agreements or guidelines around unacceptable behaviour. These actions should include the input of the nurses, multidisciplinary team, and patient as much as possible. We have also learned the importance of inviting staff members in less privileged positions to take part in safely feeding back the outcomes of interventions put in place to minimise the experience of racist and other discriminatory behaviours. This is likely to aid the team and/or department in developing best practice in managing harmful discriminatory behaviours and effectively supporting all staff involved.

Conclusion

The importance of developing a shared understanding when working with patients is vital. Research has highlighted the link between the team formulation and patient care. Furthermore, the ability for a team to explore the impact of the social and contextual factors on patient care cannot be underestimated. The reflective practice models highlighted above demonstrate contained and safe ways for this exploration to take place in the neurorehabilitation context. Additionally, these psychological frames can be a useful aid for neuropsychologists to attend to inequalities and experiences of discrimination against members of staff with protected characteristics. Furthermore, the neuropsychologist can use these tools to assist the service in developing best practice in managing harmful discriminatory behaviours and effectively supporting all staff involved.

References

Berry, K., Barrowclough, C., & Wearden, A. (2009). A Pilot Study Investigating the Use of Psychological Formulations to Modify Psychiatric Staff Perceptions of Service Users with Psychosis. *Behavioural and Cognitive Psychotherapy, 37,* 39–48. DOI: 10.1017/S1352465808005018.

Birdsey, N., & Kustner, C. (2020). Reviewing the Social GRACES: What Do They Add and Limit in Systemic Thinking and Practice? *The American Journal of Family Therapy, 49*(5), 429–442.

Bowen, A., James, M., & Young, G. (2016). *Royal College of Physicians 2016 National Clinical Guideline for Stroke* (5th ed). RCP.

Burnham, J. (1992). Approach, Method, Technique: Making Distinctions and Creating Connections. *Human Systems: The Journal of Systemic Consultation and Management, 3*(1), 3–26.

Burnham, J. (2018). Developments in Social GRRRAAACCEEESSS: Visible-invisible and voiced-unvoiced 1. In I.-B. Krause (Ed.), *Culture and Reflexivity in Systemic Psychotherapy* (pp. 139–160). Routledge.

Burnham, J., Palma, D., & Whitehouse, L. (2008). Learning as a context for differences and differences as a context for learning. *Journal of Family Therapy, 30,* 529–542. DOI: 10.1111/j.1467–6427.2008.00436.x.

Butler, C. (2015). Intersectionality in family therapy training: Inviting students to embrace the complexities of lived experience. *Journal of Family Therapy, 37*(4), 583–589.

Christofides, S., Johnstone, L., & Musa, M. (2012). 'Chipping in': Clinical psychologists' descriptions of their use of formulation in multidisciplinary team working. *Psychology and Psychotherapy: Theory, Research and Practice, 85*(4), 424–435.

Cole, S., Wood, K., & Spendelow, J. (2015). Team formulation: A critical evaluation of current literature and future research directions. *Clinical Psychology Forum, 275,* 13–18.

Craven-Staines, S., Dexter-Smith, S., & Li, K. (2010). Integrating psychological formulations into older people's Service – three years on (Part 3): Staff perceptions of formulation meetings. *PSIGE Newsletter, 112,* 16–22.

Crenshaw, K. (1991). Mapping the Margins: Intersectionality, Identity Politics, and Violence against Women of Color. *Stanford Law Review, 43*(6), 1241–1299.

Crowe, M., Carlyle, D., & Farmar, R. (2008). Clinical formulation for mental health nursing practice. *Journal of Psychiatric and Mental Health Nursing, 15*(10), 800–807.

Department of Health. (2005, March). *National Service Framework for Long-term Conditions*. Retrieved December 30, 2021, from https://assets. publishing.service.gov.uk/government/uploads/system/uploads/ attachment_data/file/198114/National_Service_Framework_for_Long_ Term_Conditions.pdf.

Dexter-Smith, S. (2007). Integrating formulations into inpatient services. *PSIGE Newsletter, 97*, 38–42.

Division of Clinical Psychology. (2011). *Good practice guidelines on the use of psychological formulation*. British Psychological Society.

Geach, N., Moghaddam, N. G., & De Boos, D. (2018). A systematic review of team formulation in clinical psychology practice: Definition, implementation, and outcomes. *Psychology and Psychotherapy: Theory, Research and Practice, 91*(2), 186–215.

Hollingworth, P., & Johnstone, L. (2014, May). Team formulation: What are the staff views. *Clinical Psychology Forum, 257*(5), 28–34.

Holmes, J. (2002). Acute wards: Problems and solutions: Creating a psychotherapeutic culture in acute psychiatric wards. *Psychiatric Bulletin, 26*, 383–385. DOI: 10.1192/pb.26.10.383.

Hood, N., Johnstone, L., & Christofides, S. (2013). The hidden solution?: Staff experiences, views and understanding of the role of psychological formulation in multi-disciplinary teams. *Journal of Critical Psychology, Counselling and Psychotherapy, 13*(2), 107–116.

Johnstone, L., & Dallos, R. (2013). *Formulation in Psychology and Psychotherapy: Making Sense of People's Problems* (2nd ed.). Routledge. DOI: 10.4324/9780203380574.

Julien, C., & Simkiss, R. (2013). Stepping up psychological care after stroke: An evaluation of psychologist and service-user led level 1 training for MDT stroke professionals. *International Journal of Stroke, 8*, 1–75.

Kerr, I., Dent-Brown, K., & Parry, G. (2007). Psychotherapy and mental health team. *International Review of Psychiatry, 19*, 63–80. DOI: 10.1080/ 09540260601109380.

Likupe, G. (2006). Experiences of African nurses in the UK National Health Service: A literature review. *Journal of Clinical Nursing, 15*, 1213–1220. DOI: 10.1111/j.1365-2702.2006.01380.x.

Miller, K. L., & Kontos, P. C. (2013). The intraprofessional and interprofessional relations of neurorehabilitation nurses: A negotiated order perspective. *Journal of Advanced Nursing, 69*(8), 1797–1807.

Moore, E., & Drennan, G. (2013). Complex forensic case formulation in recovery-oriented services: Some implications for routine practice. *Criminal Behaviour and Mental Health: CBMH, 23*, 230–240. DOI: 10.1002/cbm.1885.

Murphy, S. A., Osborne, H., & Smith, I. (2013). Psychological consultation in older adult inpatient settings: A qualitative investigation of the impact on staff's daily practice and the mechanisms of change. *Aging & Mental Health, 17*(4), 441–448.

Nolte, L. (2017). (Dis)gracefully navigating the challenges of diversity learning and teaching: Reflections on the social graces as a diversity training tool. *Context, 151*(1), 4–6.

Pearce, W. B., & Cronen, V. E. (1980). *Communication, action, and meaning: The creation of social realities*. Praeger.

Rainforth, M., & Laurenson, M. (2014). A literature review of case formulation to inform mental health practice. *Journal of Psychiatric and Mental Health Nursing, 21*(3), 206–213.

Reder, P., & Fredman, G. (1996). The Relationship to Help: Interacting Beliefs about the Treatment Process. *Clinical Child Psychology and Psychiatry, 1*(3), 457–467. DOI: 10.1177/1359104596013012.

Roper-Hall, A. (1998). Working systemically with older people and their families who have 'come to grief'. In P. Sutcliffe, G. Tufnell, & U. Cornish (Eds.), *Working with the dying and bereaved: Systemic approaches to therapeutic work.* Macmillan.

Sue, D. W., Capodilupo, C. M., Torino, G. C., Bucceri, J. M., Holder, A., Nadal, K. L., & Esquilin, M. (2007). Racial microaggressions in everyday life: Implications for clinical practice. *American Psychologist, 62*(4), 271–286.

Summers, A. (2006). Psychological formulations in psychiatric care: Staff views on their impact. *Psychiatric Bulletin, 30,* 341–343. DOI: 10.1192/pb.30.9.341.

Taylor, K. N., & Sambrook, S. (2012). CBT for culture change: Formulating teams to improve patient care. *Behavioural and Cognitive Psychotherapy, 40*(4), 496–503.

Wainwright, N., & Bergin, L. (2010). Introducing psychological formulations in an acute older people's inpatient mental health ward: A service evaluation of staff views. *PSIGE Newsletter, 112,* 38–45.

Wilson, B. A., & Betteridge, S. (2019). *Essentials of neuropsychological rehabilitation.* Guilford Publications.

Wood, K. (2016). *Clinical psychologists' experiences of moving towards using team formulation in multidisciplinary settings.* University of Surrey. https://openresearch.surrey.ac.uk/discovery/delivery/44SUR_INST:44SUR_VU1/12139808660002346.

3 Using the Tree of Life in Brain Injury Contexts

An Invitation to Accessible and Culturally Sensitive Practices

Amanda Mwale, Claire F. Whitelock, Ndidi Boakye and Camille Julien

The Foundations of the 'Tree of Life' and the Rights to Authorship of Life

The Tree of Life (ToL) methodology is a community therapeutic approach that has its foundations in Narrative Therapy, which encourages safe, empowering, and culturally sensitive storytelling (Ncube, 2006). Narrative approaches advocate for therapists to be 'decentred' in their practice. This places the individual seeking help and their social context, culture, stories, history, skills, knowledges, and rituals at the centre (Ncube, 2006; Denborough, 2014). In addition, narrative practitioners are encouraged to take an 'influential' position, which does not impose one's own personal agenda and socio-political lens (Ilic, 2017). Instead, thoughtful questions and reflections are used by the influential therapist to provide the necessary building blocks and scaffolding to support a person to maintain their 'primary authorship status' in addressing the problems and concerns of their lives.

Narrative approaches aim to take a critical look at the totalising, oppressive, and marginalising narratives in people's lives, which may have been imposed by specific institutions, histories, legacies, and socio-cultural contexts. An example includes exploration of ongoing systemic racism or ableism contributing to people's experiences of oppressive treatment by individuals and public services. Narrative therapy seeks to explore and thicken the individuals' more empowering alternative stories that recognise skills, abilities, contributions, valued relationships, and competencies. When the authorship rights are given back to the individual seeking help, this powerfully reaffirms their life and preferred identity. It also demonstrates how they have been able to utilise their own unique set of characteristics to resist the influence of their difficulties on their lives (White et al., 1990; White, 2003).

ToL was originally developed in response to the trauma, loss, and hardships faced by vulnerable children who had been orphaned as a result of

DOI: 10.4324/9781003309819-5

HIV and AIDS in Southern Africa (Ncube, 2006). This approach pro-vided an 'Island of Safety' from which children could metaphorically 'stand' and begin to talk about the 'storms' of their lives without the risk of re-traumatisation. Since its development, the ToL has been adapted within a variety of contexts to support people to reconnect with their strengths, values, hopes, and preferred identity. Adaptations of the ToL have been made in inpatient mental health settings (Wellman, Lepori, & Szlachcic, 2016) along with individuals experiencing bipolar (Ibrahim & Allen, 2018) and anorexia nervosa (Ibrahim & Tchanturia, 2018). The approach has also been adopted in physical health contexts, such as supporting children living with diabetes (Jain & MacQueen, 2021) and supporting parents with physically unwell children (Haselhurst et al., 2021). ToL has also been used to support families to adjust to the conse-quences of brain injury (e.g., Butera-Prinzi, Charles, & Story, 2014).

When the ToL methodology is applied, individuals are often intro-duced to the idea of a tree as a metaphor for their lives, with its parts representing different elements (Ncube, 2006; Haselhurst et al., 2021). See Table 3.1 for a summary of what each element on the tree represents:

All the above elements of the ToL aim to explore precious memories, hopes, experiences, skills, perspectives, and valued relationships. After richly describing their tree, participants are then invited to explore how they might respond to incoming 'storms', which represent the difficulties and challenges in their lives (Ncube, 2006).

Narrative approaches such as the ToL remove the requirement to be well accustomed to mainstream individualised Western psychological ideas and constructs, such as descriptions of diagnosable 'disorders' or reference to the decontextualised 'self' (Thomas, 2002; Ingle, 2021).

Table 3.1 The Tree of Life Metaphor

Roots	Represent an individual's history, culture and any stories relevant to their family of origin, early memorable experiences (e.g. favourite song, dance, sayings, family 'motto' or values) and important or memorable places.
Ground	Represents what activities people are engaged in currently, in their lives, which includes where they live, what they enjoy doing in their spare time and with whom they spend their time.
Trunk	Represents skills, abilities and competencies
Branches	Represent a future orientated stance, which asks individuals to talk about their hopes, dreams and wishes.
Leaves	Represent important people to the individual. These can include people who have inspired or influenced them even if they have never met, as well as those that may no longer be alive.
Fruits	Represent gifts that the individual has received from others, which may be non-physical gifts such as generosity, compassion and love
Flowers	Represent the gifts or contributions that the individual has offered to others.

Multicultural people of the global majority accessing therapeutic health services may feel alienated by these approaches, which dominate mainstream healthcare (Ingle, 2021). We use the term *global majority* here to refer to people of colour, Black, and indigenous people who comprise the majority of the world, who nonetheless hold less power and experience persisting inequalities (Lee et al., 2021). Using ToL honours and contextualises unique understandings about people's well-being and identity by taking an interest in their country of origin, culture, community, history, and socio-economic circumstances.

ToL and Brain Injury

There is increasing awareness of the usefulness of narrative approaches in the context of neurorehabilitation due to the way in which brain injury can challenge identity and sense of self (e.g., Butera-Prinzi, Charles, & Story, 2014; Hawkins, Eggleston, & Brown, 2019). Narrative practices support adjustment to living with a brain injury through reconnecting affected individuals with their history, culture, values, loved ones, skills, contributions, hopes, and dreams. In practice, we also recognised that using the ToL in brain injury can be more accessible than using talking-only methods. This is because it reduces language demands and does not rely heavily on memory or literacy skills. It is also creative and thus can support easier rapport development and co-construction of the therapeutic conversation between practitioner and the individual. The emphasis on creating a visual tree and reflecting on one's life might possibly offer a slower pace during the rehabilitation experience, with reduced demands and expectations. This might contrast the pace of physical exercises, medical reviews, assessments, clinical interviews, and the experience of being a recipient of 'education' about one's brain injury. This approach also allows for 'decentred and influential' practice (Ilic, 2017). This means that a 'patient' becomes a person who is central to describing and authoring their lives.

Our 'Tree of Intent': Preparing Our Ground for ToL Work in Brain Injury

For all clinicians and therapists considering using ToL methodology in their work in brain injury, we strongly encourage the creation of a Tree of Intent as a starting point. This process supported us in responding to the initial 'storms' we came across in starting this work ourselves. Claire, Ndidi, and I (Amanda) came together a few years ago to share our interest in starting ToL work with inpatients who had experienced a stroke in our neurorehabilitation service. The Tree of Intent was created as a means of informing and enriching our practice. It was a collective effort, developed to clarify our hopes, wishes, intentions, and the values that underpinned our shared interest in introducing the approach to our therapeutic practices.

Prior to commencing ToL approaches, our work with stroke survivors in group settings predominantly drew upon cognitive behavioural therapy ideas, which were guided by Western psychological theories of psychological disorder and individualistic recovery. We also utilised established models of 'grief' and 'psychological adjustment'. These ways of working offered 'psychoeducation' and cognitive 'techniques' to manage 'unhelpful' thoughts and ease painful emotions. Given these experiences, we were aware of the potential to unintentionally drift into 'centred influential practice', in which we assume more of an expert position in response to patients' difficulties. We therefore anticipated the Tree of Intent would act as an anchor that we returned to regularly to support ongoing reflection and reflexivity in our unfolding ToL practices. We also aimed to use the Tree of Intent to richly expand our collective narratives about the progression of the work. This includes how we made sense of the outcomes, how we evaluated the work and its potential, as well as how we thoughtfully navigated the changes and adaptations that were needed within an acute hospital setting.

The Tree of Intent initially started out as emerging ideas and energy. We then decided to physically portray this using the ToL format. See Figure 3.1 below for an example of the first drawing of our Tree of Intent.

The process of talking through the different parts of the Tree of Intent supported the motivation, energy, and enthusiasm to embark on the work. The metaphor served as our own 'island of safety' in the work. The roots depicted our educational, family, and cultural backgrounds. A mixture of Zimbabwean, Nigerian, and British heritage supported our 'roots', which were embedded in valuing difference and diversity as well as wisdom through legacy. Our clinical psychology training backgrounds and institutions were represented, recognising the opportunities they offered in supporting development of reflective practices. Further training in systemic practice was highlighted due to the way in which it privileged 'context' to be at the heart of understanding the human experience. We also considered the richness of our heritages and the stories within them. Our commitment to social justice was also discussed. The ground represented where we were conducting our work – in South London within a multicultural neurorehabilitation service. Our collective trunk represented the stories of our pre-existing skill set and how these might support us to embark on work using the ToL. These skills included technical knowledge about brain injury as well as the ability to adapt therapeutic approaches with individuals where, for example, difficulties with cognition and physical disability were present. The branches represented our collective hopes in conducting the work. This included offering survivors of a brain injury an 'Island of Safety' from which they could navigate the complexities of rehabilitation and life beyond it. We also hoped for a paradigm shift and

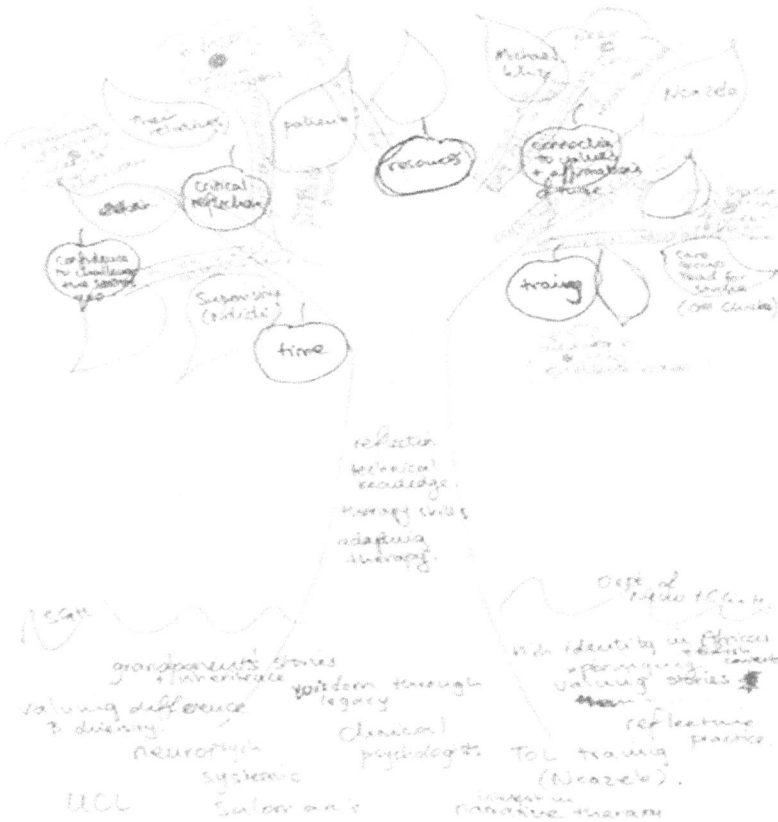

Figure 3.1 The First Drawing of the 'Tree of Intent'

an alternative approach to Structural psychological models of adjustment and well-being after brain injury. The fruits represented a variety of 'gifts' from people who have supported our interest in systemic and narrative approaches, and the flowers represented what we have been able to contribute and offer to others. This included creative insights offered to fellow clinicians in team meetings as well as adding to the limited evidence base through our practices of ToL in the brain injury clinical setting.

We also used the Tree of Intent to anchor reflections about the challenges or 'storms' we came up against in implementing the ToL group approach in a busy and sometimes unpredictable ward environment. More discussions on adaptations and adjustments are demonstrated using case examples within this chapter. The most important experience that arose from exploring our Tree of Intent was the collective support we offered each other as clinicians embarking on uncharted territory for ourselves and the service. We valued the ongoing sharing of ideas and learning from the work that seemed to break barriers across diverse intersections of culture, socio-economic circumstances, education, gender, age, ethnicity, health status, and disability.

ToL Groups in the Inpatient Neurorehabilitation Context

People with brain injury often tell us (or are invited to tell us) about what they have lost: valued abilities, roles, and skills; self-esteem; and wished-for futures (e.g., de Haan et al., 1993; Jumisko, Lexell, & Soderberg, 2005). Within and through these stories, survivors can report a felt sense of confusion about their 'place' in life (von Mensenkampff et al., 2015): both in relation to other people (How do others view me now?) and in relation to the self (Who am I now?).

We have found that the ToL model holds great value as a group intervention in the brain injury context, and it is one which we believe touches on several important themes within the process of rehabilitation: the reconnection with or reconstruction of identity and social relationships, and the generation of hope and confidence in moving forward in life despite often very significant experiences of loss and trauma. One recent example, a Hong Kong-based randomised control trial, suggests that stroke survivors participating in a narrative therapy group intervention reported significantly better outcomes in terms of their sense of meaning in life, self-mastery, self-esteem, and life satisfaction than those participating in a purely psycho-educational group (Chow, 2018). In using the ToL, problem-saturated accounts of brain injury and its consequences, which can result in survivors feeling defined by loss or disability (Morris, 2004), are respectfully challenged, whilst alternative, preferred, and richer self-narratives, which capture the person around the problem, are thickened (Ncube, 2006).

In addition, within the group setting, further elements of narrative practice underlying the tree can be explored, including the use of 'outsider witness' of group members' preferred stories by other members: further strengthening the preferred self-narratives and commitments. Having life-affirming self-narratives witnessed by others is important when considering that both problems and identities are formed in relation to other people and to the wider system (White et al., 1990). Group practices also recognise the importance of the collective for recovery (Denborough, 2012). Group members are invited to 'plant' their individual trees together as a visual 'forest', before attention turns to generating solutions for the problems facing them (Ncube, 2006). The facilitator attempts to connect the narratives of each group member through retelling stories of the forest using shared language, values, and hopes. This can provide a sense of a community 'standing together' against the storms of brain injury (White et al., 1990). Individual resources and wisdoms are shared amongst the collective and support is gained from others, thus encouraging a collaborative approach to problem-solving, which can act to challenge the sense of isolation often experienced by brain injury survivors (e.g., Schwarzberg, 1994; von Mensenkampff et al., 2015). Furthermore, in several cultures a group or relational approach to problem-solving can have much greater resonance than therapeutic practices (or rehabilitation goals) that privilege individualism and independence (Denborough, 2012).

Our Experience of the Challenges and Opportunities of ToL Groups in Brain Injury

Typically, ToL groups are conducted as single-day workshops or across several shorter sessions and can be up to eight hours in total. However, when using this approach on both an acute stroke rehabilitation unit and an inpatient neurorehabilitation unit, we were challenged to think flexibly about how to make the group accessible to as many 'patients' as possible and how to fit practically with the workings of the ward environments.

Shortening the time taken to between four and six one-hour slots fit more readily with ward timetabling requirements and reduced demands on group members' levels of fatigue, attention, and cognitive processing. The structure encompassed all four elements of the group method described by Ncube (2006), however we often added additional sessions or combined contents from different sessions according to the pacing and practical needs (e.g., upcoming discharge, medical instability) of each group cohort (see Table 3.2). In some cases, we offered additional one-to-one sessions with group members outside of the group to allow them the time to finish constructing their tree, or to prepare notes on how they wished to share their story prior to sharing this with the wider group.

We noticed that people with more severe cognitive or language impairment were more likely to be excluded from local therapeutic groups and more likely to be 'spoken for' by others within their rehabilitation. It was important to us in using the ToL that we allowed opportunities to 'give voice' to every 'patient'. In order to achieve this, we used written and visual aids, including guidelines, prompts, and examples of trees from previous groups (with permission) and our own lives, which provided an anchor for ourselves and group members in navigating the tree metaphor when more abstract concepts within it felt difficult to grasp. We provided resources from which members could select or draw inspiration, including pre-drawn tree templates and cards containing common choices for skills, fruits, and flowers. When group members had great difficulty telling us about themselves, perhaps as a result of expressive aphasia, we sought permission to access information about them from their medical records, family, and other professionals, which was then 'vetted' by the individual for inclusion (or not) on their tree. There is more on adapting the ToL for participant groups exclusively with aphasia later in this chapter.

Table 3.2 Session Structure for Brain Injury ToL Groups

Session Number(s)	Topic	Activities
1 to 2	Drawing Our Trees	Introduction to the Tree metaphor and the group aims; collective 'group rule' setting. Group members draw individual Trees of Life according to prompts outlined earlier in this chapter.
2 or 3	Sharing Our Stories	Group members are invited to share their self-stories using the Tree as a guide. The facilitator asks questions intended to thicken the preferred narrative. The co-facilitator(s) takes notes on stories shared.
3 or 4* *session may be combined with Sharing Our Stories	Forest of Life	Invitation to reflect on the similarities and differences between the trees when placed together as a 'Forest.' The facilitator weaves the individual trees together using members' own language and according to the notes taken in the previous session. Members are invited to comment on what has struck them about others' stories.
4 or 5* *session may be combined with Forest of Life	The Storms of Brain Injury	With reference to the Forest as a 'safe place from which to stand', the group is encouraged to think about how they may use their skills, abilities, and resources to respond to the challenges they are facing. Ideas are collected together visually by the facilitator.
5 or 6*	Celebration & Invitation to Others	Certificate-giving 'ceremony' in which group members' commitments and identities are acknowledged and reinforced. Subsequent group or individual sessions may invite important others to hear group members' stories, view the Forest, and/or contribute to identity stories and problem-solving.

(Based on guidance in Ncube, 2006)

We rallied support from Assistant and Trainee Psychologists to provide individualised scaffolding for group members who might benefit from this. This included support with distractibility, attention difficulties, writing, and drawing as well as extra assistance understanding the tree metaphor and generating material for individual trees. There were several opportunities to support memory throughout the programme: through the use of the written/visual tree itself, the facilitated group 're-telling' during the Forest of Life, during the 'Storms of Brain Injury' and, finally, in the Celebration and certificate-giving at the end of the group. The latter acted as both a therapeutic document (Morgan, 2000) and a longer-term memory aid or summary of the identity story, commitments, and problem-solving that had been shared.

As previously mentioned, when group members required assistance to tell their stories to the group, the method was negotiated collaboratively through additional one-to-one psychology sessions, which might involve a facilitator speaking on their behalf to pre-agreed themes. Sometimes, we were provided with the opportunity to share our values in narrative ways of working with the wider MDT, whilst also benefiting from colleagues' expertise in facilitating participation (such as through consultation with Speech and Language Therapists on supported communication strategies).

As Amanda and I (Claire) reflected on our experience of running ToL groups, we acknowledged the times when we had felt challenged by adapting the model in a way that felt faithful to its intents within the neurorehabilitation inpatient context and the powerful medicalised systems in which we work. There was a 'pull' to prioritise the solving of very real emotional, cognitive, and physical problems faced by our group members and to frame the work within the language of individualised 'goals' and measurable rehabilitation 'progress'. We were also not able to generate quantitative 'evidence' to show the effectiveness of our early groups. Despite this, we were struck by how taking part in the groups had given us a less problem-saturated view of our work with brain injury. We were helped to appreciate more fully the people we were working with and were invited to decline the position of experts responsible for 'fixing' group members' lives (Morgan, 2000). In fact, we found that the rebuilding of connections to members' own resources and aspirations sometimes resulted in previously unexplored avenues (or goals) opening up within their rehabilitation journey, both for the individual in question and ourselves. And it is upon those 'sparkling moments' (Morgan, 2002) that we continue to build our story in this way of working.

Couple ToL (CTOL)

In 2009, Wakhungu (Denborough, 2009) initiated the use of the ToL for couples but maintained an individual structure of the construction of the tree. Chimpén-López, Pacheco, Pretel-Luque, Bastón, and Chimpén-Sagrado (2021) developed the application further, reinforcing the identity and strengths of the couple by encouraging them to remember what they value about each other and to make visible their values. The first part in the intervention involves the development of the various components of the couple's identities using the metaphor of a tree. Each member of the couple draws their individual tree (roots, land, trunk, branches, leaves, and fruits) and then shares with their partner the stories that emerged during the making of it. The construction of the tree and the ensuing conversation allows couples to reconnect through their local knowledge. Alternative relational stories are developed in a safe territory where the couple can face problems, re-examine them, and strengthen themselves using the resources they have. This approach allows for the creation of a single tree for each couple, which then offers a means to reconstruct and strengthen the couple's collective identity and, in turn, the personal identity of each member.

In the second part, the couples are asked to draw a single tree representative of their relationship and to write and talk about each component. For the roots, the couple discuss the people who taught them something meaningful as a couple, and they may choose their favourite place and or their favourite song. On the ground of the CTOL, they are asked to talk about some of the common activities they do and where they live now. On reaching the trunk, the couple reflect on the values, principles, abilities, and skills that distinguish them as a pair and that are common to both of them. The same is done with the branches, but here they talk about their dreams, expectations, and desires as a couple. The leaves represent the people who are important to the couple. Finally, the fruits are the material or emotional gifts that other people offer them. Chimpén-López et al. (2021) state that some couples drew birds' nests or flowers on their CTOL. In this case, both elements represent the gifts that the couple have given to other people.

In the third part of the CTOL, the aim is to create a space of collective security in a group setting. To do so, *The Couple's Forest of Life* is built by putting trees created by each couple together in one place in the room, which ensures a communal and non-hostile territory. From that place, each couple's drawing is shared with all the participants, and a retelling of each part of the collective tree is proposed after listening to each couple's stories.

The final part of the CTOL is *The Storms of the Couple's Life*, i.e., the dangers or possible problems with which the couples may be or have been troubled. Here, the couples examine their strengths, focus on their capacities, and identify their skills and knowledge. This discussion also enables the couples to recognise how much they value their relationship, their experiences, and their collective identity. Chimpén-López et. (2021) highlighted that, when doing the final part of the CTOL, the group itself, rather than the therapist, offers alternatives to problems, suggests new possibilities, and establishes connections between the participants, which favours creating a sense of community.

CTOL and Brain Injury

The strengthening of a couple's identity following a long-term condition, sickness, or traumatic life event is paramount if the couple is to be supported to stay together. Often after a brain injury, the individual with the brain injury is so focused on recovery that other members of the family or friends are forced to reorganise themselves around that individual and take on new roles. Furthermore, moderate or severe brain injury can result in different types of disabilities (cognitive, emotional, and behavioural), which in turn can affect intimate relationships. It is not uncommon for partners to feel that 'this is not the person I know or married'. Poor marital adjustment, greater financial strain, a distancing of previously shared interests, redistribution of roles, increased dependence on partners, increased levels of stress and burden, and reduced emotional well-being, including clinically significant levels of anxiety and depression, are commonly reported (Backhaus et al., 2016; Godwin et al., 2011; O'Keeffe et al. 2020). The use of the CTOL to support couples to reinforce their identity and strengths in the context of brain injury has not yet been explored. However, there is some anecdotal evidence that this methodology can be useful in brain injury.

Case Example

Cassie and Bob were a White, British, working-class couple, aged 67 and 73 years old respectively. Cassie was diagnosed with Progressive Ataxic Syndrome (affecting the cerebella) five years into their retirement. Furthermore, after the national COVID-19 pandemic, Cassie had become progressively worse. She had initially only been able to walk short distances before needing to use her wheelchair, but now she was unable to speak without using an assistive aid and was confined to her wheelchair. Cassie also had limited use of her limbs. She was wholly dependent on Bob to feed her and carry out her personal care. Bob was severely depressed; on the Patient Health Questionnaire-9, his score was 18. He reported feelings of depression and disappointment with himself when he lost his temper whilst carrying out personal care for Cassie. He described himself as abrasive in tone. He grieved openly for the life they used to have and the plans they had for their retirement. In their first session, the couple drew their individual trees. Cassie's tree was drawn by her psychologist under her guidance.

It was difficult at first to get Bob to discuss his hopes and the gifts he felt he had been given. He seemed stuck in a problem-saturated story about the impact of ataxia on their lives. However, as the sessions progressed, the use of the tree as a metaphor enabled him to access his values (principles of life) and communicate them. He drew their CTOL (Figure 3.2) with guidance from Cassie.

For example, Bob found that loyalty was a strong value for him and Cassie, and as a result, it influenced the fruits they had been given by others in their life.

The storm of life (Ataxia) had allowed the couple to 'be cared for' and 'loved' by friends and family. Bob discovered he had developed more skills: he now was able to cook and was viewed by Cassie as her 'super-hero'. This allowed a therapeutic repair of the view he had of himself as disappointing her when he was fatigued from caring for her. They both also discovered that Ataxia wasn't always present in their lives, which

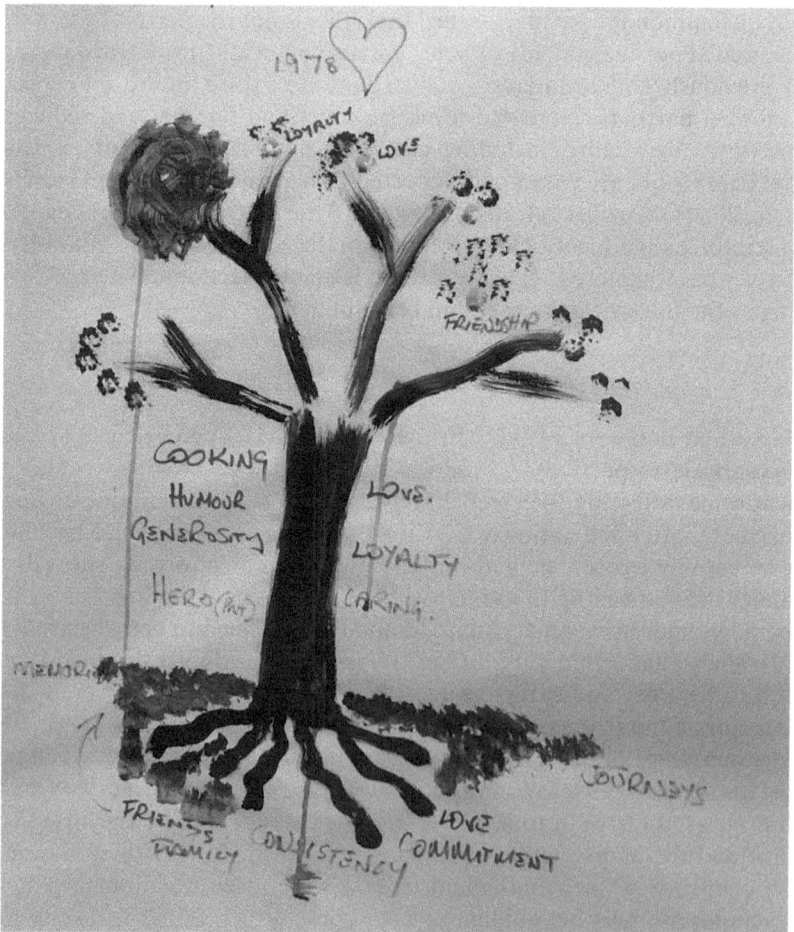

Figure 3.2 CTOL

they were surprised by, and they still had a lot of hope. Towards the end of the sessions, when sharing their story with the other members of the MDT (who acted as witnesses to their story), the couple reported that CTOL enabled them to talk more, rather than just sit in front of the television. They rediscovered the values they shared as a couple and the activities they enjoyed, such as laughing and joking together.

ToL in Aphasia

Background to the ICAP 'ToL' Group

As part of my role as neuropsychologist on a new intensive comprehensive aphasia programme (ICAP), I (Camille) was tasked with designing and setting up a psychological therapy programme for people living with aphasia and their families. This included neuropsychological assessment, therapeutic individual and group interventions, family intervention, and consultation to the speech and language therapy team on the ICAP. The ICAP ran for three weeks, with cohorts of three to four people with aphasia attending speech therapy and psychology on a day-patient basis, Monday to Friday, for up to seven hours a day (Leff et al., 2021). I will focus here on the group intervention component of the psychology programme.

From my own clinical experience and from reading the literature, I was acutely aware of the devastating impact that aphasia can have on individuals' sense of identity as well as the many barriers faced by people with aphasia when accessing talking therapy. The experience of living with aphasia has previously been likened to 'identity theft' (Shadden, 2005), with individuals describing a profound sense of disconnection from previous strengths, abilities, and values, leading to disrupted 'biographic narratives' and a sense of self as 'incompetent' (Baker et al., 2020; D'Cruz, Douglas, & Seery, 2019). With a fragmented sense of self no longer able to support full participation in life and relationships, people with aphasia are at greater risk of experiencing reduced quality of life, social isolation, and mood disturbances (Clarke & Black, 2005; Hilari et al., 2012). A group intervention that used a strengths-based narrative therapy approach therefore seemed a unique opportunity to bring people together and draw on collective resources to support individuals to rebuild a coherent, integrated sense of identity. The ToL framework, with its highly visual and structured format, seemed well suited to supporting the cognitive and communication needs of people with aphasia. As the ICAP brought together individuals from all over the UK with diverse ethnic, socioeconomic, and cultural backgrounds, it offered a simple and elegant way to understand the unique cultural, historical, and socio-economic aspects of individuals' contexts that contributed to identity and well-being.

Running the Group

The group ran for two hours a week over the three weeks of the ICAP and was held in a large outpatient room in a hospital setting. It was facilitated by a clinical psychologist and a trainee psychologist. A ratio of one facilitator to two clients was required to enable facilitation of oral and written communication. Tailored communication and cognitive supports were developed based on speech therapy and psychology recommendations for maximising client engagement with therapeutic interventions (e.g., the facilitator drawing or writing on behalf of the client; using written options to facilitate verbal generation). Table 3.3 provides an outline of each group session.

Case Example

Grace was a 56-year-old woman who had suffered a left middle cerebral artery infarct 12 months earlier, which left her with moderate expressive aphasia and right-sided weakness. She originated from Ghana and had moved to the UK at the age of 26 to join her husband. They had five children and subsequently separated when Grace was in her 40s. As well as raising her children, Grace held a range of jobs, including hairdresser, cleaner, and 'dinner lady'. She had a strong Christian faith and had built up a solid social network around her work and church. Following the stroke, she was no longer able to work and, although she still attended

Table 3.3 Session Outline for the ICAP ToL Group

Session 1: The ToL	See box 2
Session 2: The forest of life	See Box 2
Session 3: The storms of aphasia	Having created a safe place of strength, ability and hope from which to stand (the riverbank position), the exercise now invites participants to talk about some of the difficulties and challenges they are experiencing as a result of their stroke and/or aphasia, in ways that are not re-traumatising. Using the metaphor of aphasia/ stroke as a storm, participants share their collective experience of living with aphasia and unpack some of the skills and abilities they have already used to cope with challenges.
	Participants are asked to reflect on gains they have made on the programme and they have seen others make. They share their hopes and goals for the next few months and identify from the tree resources, skills and people who will help them achieve their goals and sustain gains.

(Adapted from Ncube, 2006)

church, she avoided speaking to people and singing in the choir, as she worried people would see her differently as a result of her communication and physical difficulties. Although she retained some contact with her children, she described a deep sense of isolation and fear of burdening others and, as a result, she experienced low mood.

As Grace was unable to hold a pen, she gave consent for the psychologist to draw and label the tree under her instruction. When tracing her roots, Grace reflected on her childhood experiences of living in a large family household in Ghana, going to church, and helping her mother sell yams in the local market. She felt these formative experiences had helped shape her into a 'sunshine' person, who willingly gave to others and flourished from making others laugh. These qualities formed the basis of her trunk – a 'funny woman' and a 'free giver' who would 'talk to anybody', 'make people laugh', and was strikingly generous: 'If you ask me and I don't have, I will go and get it for you'. She also expressed pride at having extricated herself from an abusive marital relationship and becoming a 'free woman'. Revisiting these strengths and past experiences of resilience helped Grace to realise that, through withdrawing from others, she had become disconnected from her sense of identity as a 'sunshine woman', and this had precipitated a sense of isolation and a decline in her mood. She used the branches of the tree to consider new ways she could reconnect with her values while living with aphasia. These included mingling with people more at church, rejoining the choir, and finding ways to help others at her local stroke club. She also had longer-term hopes of going to college to improve her English and find work again. Sharing her tree with other members of her cohort was a powerful experience for Grace and helped cement her intentions for her new life. These goals were integrated into Grace's therapy programme, and the ICAP team supported her to make contact with her church choir and develop strategies to facilitate having confident conversations with friends at church and in her local community. At follow-up three months after the programme, Grace was still singing in her choir and had started volunteering as a befriender in her local stroke club. She described feeling more confident, brighter in mood, and thrilled to have rediscovered her 'sunshine self'.

Using the ToL in Group Supervision of Nursing Staff in Neurorehabilitation

The occupational stress and strain experienced by staff nurses is well documented (Lambert & Lambert, 2001). Nursing staff in the UK are also amongst the clinical groups most exposed to violent and aggressive behaviour in their frontline caring roles (Winstanley & Whittington, 2004). Group supervision for nurses is important in providing shared learning and mutual support (Jones, 2003). As demonstrated in previous sections, the ToL can be helpfully applied to the clinical setting, within groups, with couples, and also for reflective and reflexive purposes (see the Tree of Intent). We have also applied it in the supervision of nurses in the neurorehabilitation setting.

We incorporated the ToL in supervision due to the often totalising problem stories that nurses can hold about the struggles they may face in their work. This includes navigating the complexity and challenges of diverse patients with neurological conditions in a fast-paced multi-disciplinary environment with high expectations and limited resources. Such challenges have a significant negative impact on staff morale and stress. In our work in providing clinical supervision to nursing teams, we also recognised the diversity of the workforce, including a broad variation in ethnicity, gender, age, culture, knowledges, and educational backgrounds. Introducing the Professional ToL (PToL) to ward nurses served to honour, value, and celebrate their diverse backgrounds (roots). We also hoped to reacquaint them with their skills and abilities, valued relationships, and important contributions in order to provide them with a more empowering alternative narrative about themselves and their colleagues in the context of a challenging work environment and the risk of burnout.

As previously highlighted, ordinarily a ToL group workshop takes approximately eight hours from commencement to ending. However, due to time limitations, an hour-long slot was used to begin to engage nurses in PToL during their usual monthly supervision time. Firstly, the nurses were asked to draw their professional trees, paying attention to the following prompts (See Table 3.4 below):

Table 3.4 Example Prompts for PToL

EXAMPLE PROMPTS FOR PROFESSIONAL TOL

Roots: How did you get into this work? What values are you living through your work?

Ground: Where do you work? What do you enjoy doing at work? What are your favourite work experiences?

Trunk: What are you good at? What are you known to be skilled at if we asked your colleagues?

Branches: What are your hopes, desires, wishes in relation to your work, both in the near and distant future?

Leaves: Who is important to you in your work? Who supports you to continue your work?

Fruits: What gifts have you received from others that enable you to do your work?

Flowers: What gifts have you given others in your work?

Ncazelo Ncube and Phola International, which provided training in adapting Tree of Life for use in professional contexts

A Summary of Experiences of the PToL

Roots: Some members of staff attending the session shared their educational and professional experiences, including previous and current roles (e.g., Deputy Ward Manager) as well as their values (e.g., keeping the ward safe; patient care; quality). Others shared their gender as well as racial and ethnic background (e.g., 'I am a Black woman working in ... the NHS', 'Caribbean', 'Jamaican heritage') as a significant part of their roots. Some also highlighted role models as being a part of 'who' supported the establishment of their 'roots' in the profession.

Ground and Trunk: Most of the nursing staff highlighted the ward that they worked in as their ground, with some emphasising the role of 'helping and assisting others' in their ground. Skills, abilities, and competencies represented by the trunk included being strong, dependable, confident, supportive, safe, relatable, kind, and patient as well as teaching students and having a 'serving heart'. Nursing staff were struck by just how much they were able to recognise the variety of individual and collective skills as a team.

Branches: Staff members spoke of the near future, which included continuing study and hoping for promotion to senior and higher-paying roles. Others also noted hopes for their lives after retirement, which included preferred location ('I'd like to retire somewhere in the sun') and good physical health at the point of retirement.

Leaves: Members of staff highlighted a combination of valued individuals that contributed to enabling or inspiring them to continue with their work. This included their patients admitted for neurorehabilitation, colleagues, as well as family and friends. Mentors and supervisors were also acknowledged as important in the highs and lows of their career journeys and day-to-day work.

Fruits and Flowers: Members of the nursing team highlighted the gifts of security, job satisfaction, compliments, professional development opportunities, and being cared for by others. A few nurses identified with appreciation the gift of 'bring a dish' day. This was an event where staff members were encouraged to bring to work a cooked meal from their country of origin to celebrate the multicultural team during festive times or to bid farewell to a valued team member. Nursing staff highlighted their contributions to others, which included their composure, kindness, smiles, cheerfulness, and the support they offered to others, including to patients, relatives, and colleagues.

Valuing the Forest: As a part of responding to storms that were represented by many of the challenges that nurses often brought to the supervision sessions (including staff shortages and managing challenging behaviour), we discussed the metaphor of the forest. We talked with the nurses about a 'forest' representing the strength and support that can be found in a team, as opposed to singular individual 'trees' that might be more vulnerable to storms.

Lively discussions concluded the session, with staff talking about how much they did not recognise their own unique strengths as well as the wider teams' strengths. As facilitators, Ndidi and I (Amanda) reflected on the change in body language at the end of the session, compared with how staff presented at the start. Initially, they looked exhausted after temporarily leaving their ward in the afternoon following supporting transfers of patients for bed rest. They also appeared puzzled by the paint brushes, coloured pencils, and paper we had placed in the group room.

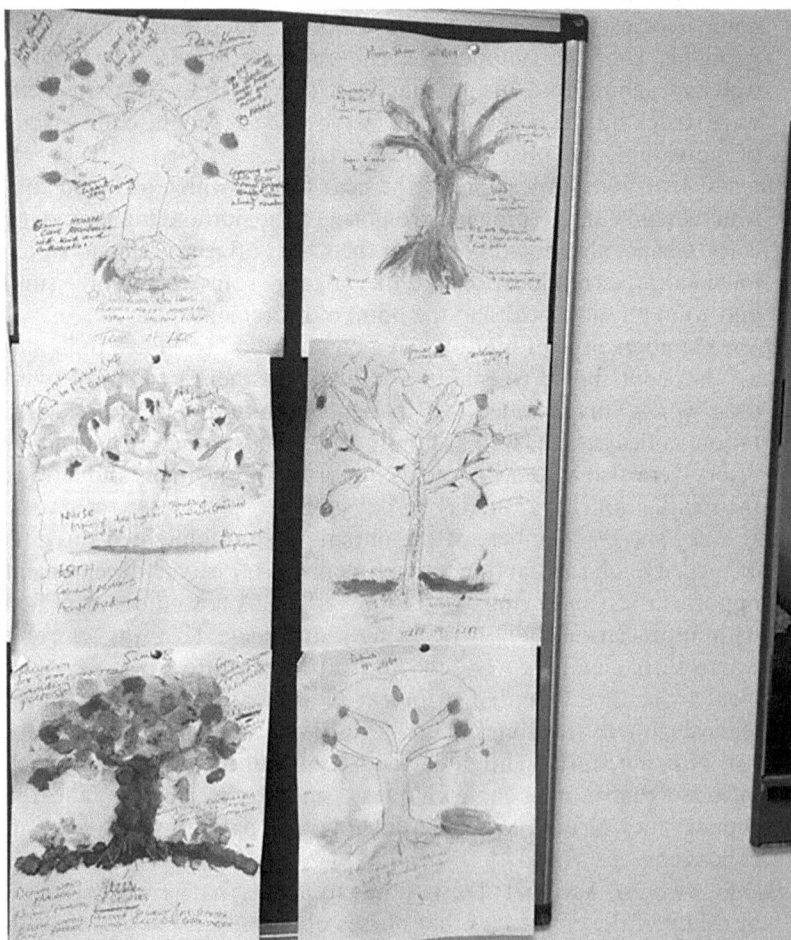

Figure 3.3 'Forest of Life' Trees Displayed in the Staff Room after PToL Session

Towards the end of the session, they were talking much more, their eye contact with each other increased, and they were laughing and sharing their drawings with each other. The nurses were keen to celebrate and share their forest with other colleagues and collectively agreed to display these in their staff room.

Our work demonstrated that PToL could be used as a useful tool to support diverse teams to recognise often neglected alternative storylines about their professional identities, skills, abilities, and contributions. The approach is culturally sensitive, allowing the individuality and intersectionality of identities to be recognised, honoured, and celebrated within a work context and amongst colleagues. PToL can be used as a method to rediscover the values, experiences, and key relationships that can be protective during challenging times working in the neurorehabilitation setting.

Chapter Summary

We hope that this chapter has demonstrated the potential breadth of the utility of ToL approaches within neurorehabilitation. It can be applied in different contexts, such as during time-limited inpatient admissions, with people with language difficulties (aphasia), with couples, and with professional teams. We strongly encourage its application and the centring of the wide variety of physical, cognitive, cultural, and educational differences that people bring to the brain injury context.

References

Backhaus, S., Neumann, D., Parrot, D., Hammond, F. M., Brownson, C., & Malec, J. (2016). Examination of an intervention to enhance relationship satisfaction after brain injury: a feasibility study. *Brain Injury, 30*(8), 975–985.

Baker, C., Worrall, L., Rose, M., & Ryan, B. (2020). 'It was really dark': The experiences and preferences of people with aphasia to manage mood changes and depression. *Aphasiology, 34*(1), 19–46.

Butera-Prinzi, F., Charles, N., & Story, K. (2014). Narrative family therapy and group work for families living with acquired brain injury. *Australian and New Zealand Journal of Family Therapy, 35*(1), 81–99.

Chimpén-López, C. A., Pacheco, M., Pretel-Luque, T., Bastón, R., & Chimpén-Sagrado, D. (2021). The couple's tree of life: Promoting and protecting relational identity. *Family Process*, 1–14. DOI: 10.1111/famp.12727.

Chow, E. O. W. (2018). Narrative group intervention to reconstruct meaning of life among stroke survivors: A randomized clinical trial study. *Neuropsychiatry, 8*(4), 1216–1226.

Clarke, P., & Black, S. E. (2005). Quality of life following stroke: Negotiating disability, identity, and resources. *Journal of Applied Gerontology, 24*(4), 319–336.

D'Cruz, K., Douglas, J., & Serry, T. (2019). Personal narrative approaches in rehabilitation following traumatic brain injury: A synthesis of qualitative research. *Neuropsychological Rehabilitation, 29*(7), 985–1004.

de Haan, R., Aaronson, N., Limburg, M., Hewer, R. L., & van Crevel, H. (1993). Measuring quality of life in stroke. *Stroke*, *24*(2), 320–327.

Denborough, D. (2009). *Alzando nuestras cabezas por encima de las nubes: el uso de las prácticas narrativas para impulsar acción social y desarrollo económico.* Dulwich Centre Foundation.

Denborough, D. (2012). A storyline of collective narrative practice: A history of ideas, social projects and partnerships. *International Journal of Narrative Therapy and Community Work*, *1*, 40–65.

Denborough, D. (2014). *Retelling the Stories of Our Lives: Everyday Narrative Therapy to Draw Inspiration and Transform Experience.* W. W. Norton & Co.

Godwin, E. E., Kreutzer, J. S., Arango-Lasprilla, J. C., & Lehan, T. J. (2011). Marriage after brain injury: Review, analysis, and research recommendations. *The Journal of Head Trauma Rehabilitation*, *26*(1), 43–55.

Haselhurst, J., Moss, K., Rust, S., ... & Murray, J. (2021). A narrative-informed evaluation of tree of life for parents of children with physical heath conditions. *Clinical Child Psychology and Psychiatry*, *26*(1), 51–63. DOI: 10.1177/1359104520972457.

Hawkins, L. G., Eggleston, D., & Brown, C. C. (2019). Utilising a narrative therapy approach with couples who have experienced a traumatic brain injury to increase intimacy. *Contemporary Family Therapy*, *41*, 304–315. DOI: 10.1007/s10591-018-9484-8.

Hilari, K., Needle, J. J., & Harrison, K. L. (2012). What are the important factors in health-related quality of life for people with aphasia?: A systematic review. *Archives of Physical Medicine and Rehabilitation*, *93*, S86–S95.

Ibrahim, J., & Allen, J. (2018). The highs and lows through recovery: An integrative group combining cognitive behavioral therapy, narrative therapy, and the tree of life. *Group*, *42*(1), 23–33. DOI: 10.13186/group.42.1.0023.

Ibrahim, J., & Tchanturia, K. (2018). Patients' experience of a narrative group therapy approach informed by the 'ToL' model for individuals with anorexia nervosa. *International Journal of Group Psychotherapy*, *68*(1), 80–91. DOI: 10.1080/00207284.2017.1315586.

Ilic, D. (2017). Conversation Analysis of Michael White's Decentered and Influential Position. PhD Dissertation. Nova Southeastern University. https://nsuworks.nova.edu/shss_dft_etd/25.

Ingle, M. (2021). Western individualism and psychotherapy: Exploring the edges of ecological being. *Journal of Humanistic Psychology*, *61*(6), 925–938.

Jain, N., & MacQueen, R. (2021). Experience of the tree of life narrative group therapy delivered virtually for children and young people with diabetes (CYPD) during COVID 19 pandemic. *Archives of Disease in Childhood*, *106*, A156. DOI: 10.1136/archdischild-2021-rcpch.271.

Jones, A. (2003). Some benefits experienced by hospice nurses from group clinical supervision. *European Journal of Cancer Care*, 12(3), 224–232. DOI: 10.1046/j.1365–2354.2003.00405.x.

Jumisko, E., Lexell, J., & Soderberg, S. (2005). The Meaning of Living with Traumatic Brain Injury in People with Moderate or Severe Traumatic Brain Injury. *Journal of Neuroscience Nursing*, *37*, 42–50.

Lambert, V. A., & Lambert, C. E. (2001). Literature review of role stress/strain on nurses: An international perspective. *Nursing & Health Sciences*, *3*, 161–172. DOI: 10.1046/j.1442–2018.2001.00086.x.

Lee, B. A., Ogunfemi, N., Neville, H. A., & Tettegah, S. (2021). Resistance and restoration: Healing research methodologies for the global majority. *Cultural Diversity and Ethnic Minority Psychology*, 1–9. DOI: 10.1037/cdp0000394.

Leff, A. P., Nightingale, S., Gooding, B., Rutter, J., Craven, N., Peart, M., ... & Crinion, J. T. (2021). Clinical Effectiveness of the Queen Square Intensive Comprehensive Aphasia Service for Patients With Poststroke Aphasia. *Stroke*, *52*(1), e594–3598. DOI: 10.1161/STROKEAHA.120.033837.

Morgan, A. (2000). *What is Narrative Therapy?: An easy to read introduction.* Dulwich Centre Publications.

Morgan, A. (2002). Beginning to use a narrative approach in therapy. *International Journal of Narrative Therapy & Community Work, 2002*(1), 85–90.

Morris, S. D. (2004). Rebuilding identity through narrative following traumatic brain injury. *Journal of Cognitive Rehabilitation*, *22*, 15–21.

Ncube, N. (2006). The ToL Project: Using narrative ideas in work with vulnerable children in Southern Africa. *International Journal of Narrative Therapy & Community Work, 2006*(1), 3–16.

O'Keeffe, F., Dunne, J., Nolan, M., Cogley, C., & Davenport, J. (2020). 'The things that people can't see': The impact of TBI on relationships: An interpretative phenomenological analysis. *Brain Injury*, *34*(4), 496–507.

Schwarzberg, S. L. (1994). Helping factors in a peer-developed support group for persons with brain injury, part 1: Participant observer perspective. *American Journal of Occupational Therapy*, *48*, 297–304.

Shadden, B. (2005). Aphasia as identity theft: Theory and practice. *Aphasiology*, *19*(3–5), 211–223.

Thomas, L. (2002). Poststructuralism and Therapy: What's It all About? *International Journal of Narrative Therapy & Community Work, 2002*(2), 85–89.

von Mensenkampff, B., Ward, M., Kelly, G., Cadogan, S., Fawsit, F., & Lowe, N. (2015). The value of normalization: Group therapy for individuals with brain injury. *Brain Injury*, *29*(11), 1292–1299.

Wellman, J., Lepori, F., & Szlachcic, R. (2016). Exploring the utility of a pilot TOL group in an inpatient setting. *The Journal of Mental Health Training, Education and Practice*, *11*(3), 172–181. DOI: 10.1108/JMHTEP-01-2016-0007.

White, M. (2003). Narrative practice and community assignments. *International Journal of Narrative Therapy and Community Work, 2003*(2), 17–55.

White, M., White, M. K., Wijaya, M., & Epston, D. (1990). *Narrative Means to Therapeutic Ends.* W. W. Norton & Co.

Whitstanley, S., & Whittington, R. (2004). Aggression towards health care staff in a UK general hospital: Variation among professions and departments. *Journal of Clinical Nursing*, *13*, 3–10. DOI: 10.1111/j.1365–2702.2004.00807.x.

4 Navigating Intersectionality in Couple Therapy for Brain Injury

Ndidi Boakye

Introduction

It is not uncommon for neuropsychologists working with couples and families to focus on single aspects of identity, e.g., disability or gender. However, it is now accepted that not attending to multiple aspects of identity when working therapeutically is problematic and can lead to poorer outcomes. Indeed, previously held assumptions in psychology about what was 'normal' or 'healthy' are now accepted to have been largely based on a White, European, heterosexual 'norm' of relationships and communication styles (Ahsan, 2020). Therapists' validation of the therapeutic relationship is essential for therapy to be successful (Eubanks, Burckell, & Goldfried, 2018). In order for a relationship to be validated, the therapist must be aware of the impact of multi-aspects of identity on couples' lived experience.

Intersectionality

The consideration of these multiple layers, identities of belonging, and how one is positioned across these is known as intersectionality. Intersectionality is a feminist theoretical concept developed from exploring the lived experience of women of colour, and the term was coined in 1989 by Kimberlé Crenshaw. The concept denotes how one is simultaneously positioned, for example, as Black, working-class, lesbian, or colonial subject (Brah & Phoenix, 2004). As such, it foregrounds a complex ontological approach that attempts to reduce people to one category at a time. It enables a lens by which the power dynamics inherent in relational systems are made visible. It is a framework for exploring many factors exerting influence on our day-to-day relationships. As clinicians, it enables us to attend to the multiple marginalised identities experienced by our patients. This is key, as when clinicians conceptualise patients from a singular lens, they may develop clinical blind spots in which crucial components of identity and context are ignored, the lived experience is missed, and therapeutic effectiveness becomes difficult to attain (Ali & Lee, 2019).

DOI: 10.4324/9781003309819-6

Intersectionality in Brain Injury

The trajectory of brain injury treatment in the UK significantly lacks consideration for intersectionality in the individuals and families living with brain injury. This is in spite of a clear understanding of brain injury as a disability that disrupts the lives of those that it touches. There is rarely a question of whose life disability is touching or the nature of the impact intersecting with other aspects of oppression. Ownsworth (2014) found that having a brain injury can alter one's sense of self or the essential qualities that define who we are. One can go from being viewed as an Asian, able-bodied, Muslim, cisgendered man already dealing with discrimination to being perceived as a disabled, Asian, Muslim, cisgendered man. There can be little awareness of the impact of disability on a life already faced with challenges. For example, what does this mean for those who want to return to work and what is the impact of this on family functioning or the couple relationship? That shift of identity and the connotations that ensue can be destabilising for our patients.

Brain Injury and the Couple Relationship

Brain injury is one example of a long-term condition that cuts across multiple identities, seemingly unifying a group under the identity of disability. However, visible aspects of identity can result in different pressures or resources for an individual living with brain injury. In the couple relationship, this is more pronounced. The experience of discrimination for couples with visible or identifiable aspects of identity is well documented (Baucom et al., 2019). For example, in the UK the social environment responds to disability with 'sympathy'. This discrimination can also be directed at the relationship, resulting in judgement or stigma. It can make it difficult for the couple to find an environment or social circle in which they feel appropriately supported.

The consequences of this can include decreased or marginalised acceptance, recognition, or validation (Baucom et al., 2019), thereby placing the relationship under great strain. In the context of brain injury, where there can be significant problems with emotional, behavioural, and cognitive functions, such as deficits in attention, learning, memory, reasoning, and decision-making, this can result in relationship strain and distress. In studies looking at the impact of brain injury on relationships, poor marital adjustment and greater financial strain are frequently reported (Backhaus et al., 2016; Bowen, Palmer, & Yeates, 2010/2018; Hammond et al., 2021; O'Keeffe et al., 2020; Stiekema et al., 2020). Further challenges to the relationship may include a distancing of previously shared interests, redistribution of roles, increased dependence on partners, reduced ability to engage in activity together, and sexual difficulties, amongst others. Increased levels of stress and burden as well as reduced emotional well-being, including clinically significant levels of anxiety and depression, have been reported by partners of people with TBI (O'Keeffe et al., 2020). Loss of empathy and sensitivity in the individual with brain injury have been highlighted as factors lowering relationship satisfaction (Godwin et al., 2011; Hammond et al., 2021). Grief and loss are central to the processes involved in adapting to living with a partner with brain injury. Klonoff (2014) suggested that these processes are compounded by the nature of the deficit and the course of recovery. If these issues are not addressed, individuals with brain injury and their partners can experience strain on their relationship.

For couples from minoritised backgrounds living with brain injury, it is important to be aware of additional pressures that they will face, such as discrimination as a result of their minority status and/or disability. It can be difficult for the individual with brain injury to get back into employment or study due to discrimination. Undue stress is therefore placed on the relationship, resulting in the partner having to carry the financial burden, work multiple jobs, or indeed not be able to perform at work due to multiple demands. There may be the additional stigma associated with having a disability or living with someone with a disability. The redistribution of roles and the impact on parenting can be difficult to negotiate. Lower-income couples may not be able to afford childcare or other needs around the home, and therefore they will be exposed to greater amounts of stress. This is in addition to other challenges, such as housing, security, worries about the family and children's future, the psychological impact of financial strain, and living in more disadvantaged neighbourhoods (Baucom et al., 2019).

Addressing Intersectionality in Treatment

It is well documented that the therapeutic alliance (i.e., the relationship between patients and clinicians) is the single common factor across treatment modality in producing positive clinical outcomes (Review of *Escape from Babel*, 1997). Therefore, the willingness and openness of neuropsychologists in addressing intersectionality with patients is likely to strengthen the therapeutic alliance, thereby positively influencing treatment outcomes (PettyJohn et al., 2020).

PettyJohn et al. (2020) suggest that clinicians can approach these conversations in a way that minimises anxiety, is sensitive to differences, and is clinically relevant. Simple statements such as this could be powerful (PettyJohn et al., 2020): 'From my Westernised therapy training, I believe [treatment approach] would be most helpful to you; however, I'd value understanding your perspective on what could be helpful, in case your experiences differ from mine.' The notion that having a conversation on intersectionality provides neuropsychologists with an opportunity to present their perspective, speak from their clinical training, provide a rationale for tasks offered, and hopefully gain buy-in from the patient is not far-fetched. Anecdotal evidence suggests that this approach leaves patients feeling understood, seen, heard, and validated. Person-centred goals will naturally flow from such an exchange. We know that therapy goals are largely impacted by how individuals have grown up, what they have experienced in life, and how they view their problems. The lens through which people perceive and process the world shapes the outcomes they see as most important (PettyJohn et al., 2020). Unsurprisingly, neuropsychologists and patients with opposing intersectional identities will have differing goals for treatment.

An example of this could be a White neuropsychologist treating a Black patient for distress related to inability to return to work and loss of his identity as a provider to his family of origin. The neuropsychologist might set their own goal of working to strengthen a new identity and identify a voluntary role for the patient in order to gain their family's support and acceptance. However, this patient (having a much more thorough understanding of their own family dynamics and beliefs about disability) may instead want to work on returning to work and reasserting himself as the 'head of the home'. While this goal may seem conflictual, a conversation with the patient will shed more light on the underlying reasons for his preferred goal, as the patient brings his own unique understanding of his family's cultural and religious beliefs. Without opening a dialogue about the intersectionality of the neuropsychologist and patient's identities, it would be difficult for either party to understand the other's perspective and work toward establishing goals that feel comfortable for the patient (PettyJohn et al., 2020). How would this work when carrying out a couple intervention? How can the neuropsychologist address the impact of socio-political factors on the couple relationship?

Behavioural Couples Therapy Treatment Model

Behavioural Couples Therapy (BCT) is a couple therapy model that takes into consideration the individual, environmental, and relational factors that impact on a couple relationship. It is therefore well suited to couples living with brain injury. It draws upon learning theory, namely the reinforcement principles of operant conditioning as well as social exchange theory (Thibaut & Kelley, 1959). Operant conditioning principles suggest that partners will be more likely to behave in positive ways towards each other if they receive positive consequences from each other for those actions (Baucom et al., 2008), whilst social exchange theory suggests that successful relationships are distinguished from unsuccessful marriages in the rate and frequency of positive reinforcements exchanged by the partners (Stuart, 1969). A scarcity of positive outcomes available for each member, particularly in relation to the frequency of negative outcomes, can consequently lead to distress within the relationship.

This approach is beneficial for couples living with brain injury, who may be adjusting to a loss of previously experienced positive outcomes and increased negative outcomes associated with changes in functioning. In BCT, the goal of the therapist is to help couples better understand their patterns of interaction and teach them relevant skill-based interventions, such as communication and decision-making. In communication skill building, for example, the pace of conversation is slowed down significantly from day-to-day styles of conversing. This encourages a positive experience of communication. Doidge (2008) suggests that therapy allows new verbal images to be made, which results in connections being drawn, which facilitates the change process. One can therefore imagine that the process of being slowed down in the communication skill building allows new verbal images of the couple in their relationship to be presented to themselves. This results in new connections made, which facilitates change. Furthermore, the process supports the mentalisation process (the ability to be both self-reflective whilst observing others and reflecting on their mental state (Lieberman, 2007)), which is thought to be disrupted in brain injury (Channon & Crawford, 2010). Other interventions include guided behaviour change (i.e., behavioural interventions that do not involve a skilled component, such as 'date nights') and cognitive restructuring. All interventions carried out are dependent on the conceptualisation of a couple's needs.

BCT Interventions to Cope with Psycho-Social Pressures

Clinicians may find themselves having to address the impact of environmental factors on the couple relationship. The interaction between external, relationship, and individual factors are shown in Figure 4.1. For example, the pressure for the individual with brain injury to return to work to alleviate financial pressures in the home.

In this example, therapy goals may include: (a) increasing the awareness and empathy of the partner with brain injury; (b) increasing individual

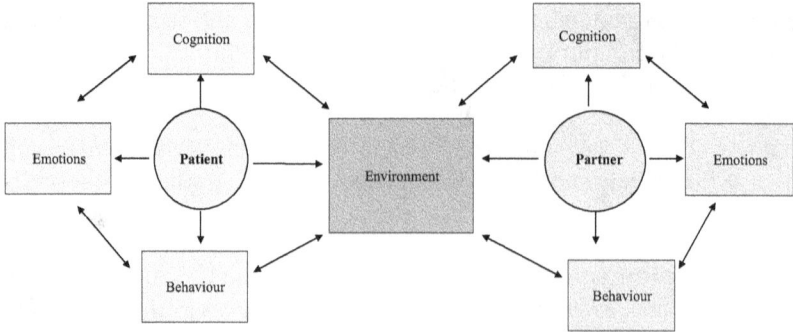

Figure 4.1 BCT Formulation Model

coping strategies for the couple; (c) communicating about the emotional impact of the situation; (d) problem-solving about the situation as a couple; and (e) increasing support. These goals can be accomplished using the sharing thoughts and feelings guidance (Table 4.1), addressing behaviour responses, and challenging cognitions.

Given the topic on intersectionality, it is important to stress that the literature in neuropsychology is overwhelmingly heteronormative: there are clearly gaps in understanding the needs of LGBTQ+ individuals within the context of brain injury. Some of these themes are addressed in Chapter 10. However, there is a call to explore this in future studies and clinically. Furthermore, in clinical practice we only see or are referred couples in monogamous relationships (the practice of marrying, cohabiting, or dating one person at a time). However, we know there are multiple models of relationships in modern society, including polyamory (having intimate relationships with more than one person at a time) and polygamy (having more than one spouse). This is another area of relatively little research, but it is important in the quest for inclusion. These relationships are not discussed in this chapter, as they are not currently part of the author's own focus of clinical experience, but there is a need to develop and understand the multiple relationships in which brain injury is experienced.

The cases about to be presented reflect couples from mixed-heritage backgrounds that the author has been privileged to have worked with for a number of years. It is worth reflecting that often these couples sought the author out based on the assumption that the cultural issues impacting the couple's relationship were more likely to be attended to. Research has long explored the role of similarity in the therapeutic process. Better outcomes have been found, which have been attributed to the therapist having a deeper understanding due to shared experiences (Atkinson, 1983; Kim & Kang, 2018). This hypothesis can be extended to couple work in brain injury. Figure 4.2 shows some of the multiple identities of the couple and the neuropsychologist intersecting in one of the case examples presented below. The two cases examples demonstrate the use of BCT interventions when working intersectionally with couples with brain injury.

Case Study One

Diaz, a 40-year-old married man with two young children, suffered a stroke at work five years ago. His wife Fleur reported that he had been low in mood since his stroke; he spent time alone away from her and the children. She described him as uninterested in them. He described her as undermining him, especially in front of their children.

Fleur was a White French female, whilst Diaz was a Black Portuguese male. Diaz had a close relationship with his parents and felt it was

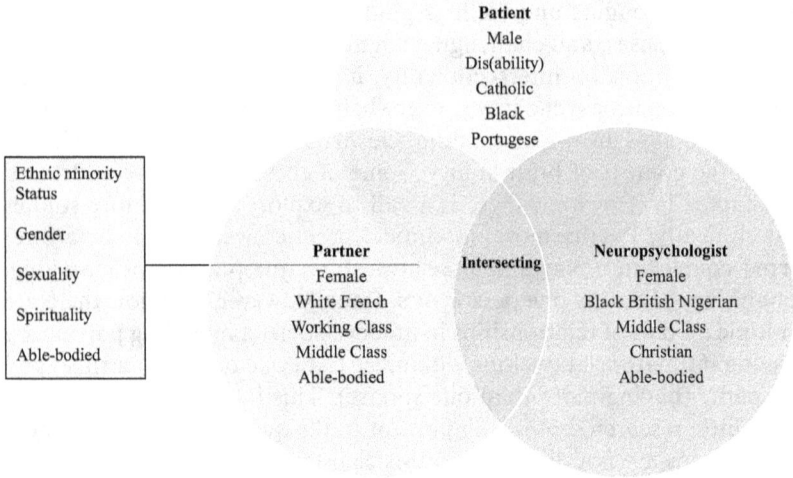

Figure 4.2 Multiple Intersecting Identities During Couple Therapy

important for them to be 'looked after'. They had raised him and invested in him over the years, and now it was 'his turn to pay back'. He wanted his children to do likewise, holding family values dear. He was keen that they be raised in a similar manner to himself with respect for elders and not 'answering back'. However, his parenting style was described by Fleur as 'authoritarian'. She felt he was 'far too hard on the kids'. On the other hand, he felt that Fleur was 'too liberal' and allowed the children to do 'anything'. Diaz's stroke left him with slower processing speed and aphasia, so he found it difficult at times to manage the children. He noticed he fatigued more quickly and withdrew to conserve his energy. Fleur found his withdrawal difficult. She felt neglected and unloved. The weight of looking after the children whilst supporting her husband, who now had a disability, was very stressful for her. It was difficult for Fleur to hold in mind Diaz's emotional and cognitive needs when she felt neglected. They found themselves arguing in front of the children, and it made them both unhappy. They decided to seek support via couple therapy.

As discussed earlier, couples can fail to recognise when their individual stressors impact the relationship and over time can become less empathetic towards each other. A therapy goal may be to help the couple to understand each other's stressors, and how stressor management impacts the other, and their overall relationship. Thus, in this case, the neuropsychologist (NB) shared the formulation regarding the standards they had about parenting and how this was shaped by their families and cultures of origin. The impact of brain injury on Diaz's behaviours, e.g., fatigue and slowed processing, was also discussed. The couple were then supported to have a conversation using the sharing thoughts and feelings guidelines (see Table 4.1). Diaz was able to communicate the impact of stroke on his life and his perceived loss of his role as parent (including raising his children in line with his cultural heritage). Fleur was surprised. She had not realised the link between his withdrawal and the stroke or how undermined he felt. She also had not considered how important it was for Diaz to raise his children as Black Portuguese. This enabled the neuropsychologist, who was Black British, to explore what their differing cultural heritages meant to them and how they influenced their parenting style. The opportunity to discuss how this intersected with disability presented itself. It was used to deliver brain injury education on the specifics of the stroke Diaz had experienced, including the psychological, cognitive, and behavioural impact. Likewise, when Fleur took the role of speaker, Diaz was surprised that his withdrawal into the bedroom was experienced as neglect of her feelings and a lack of interest. This conversation, which took place over three sessions, opened up the opportunity for the couple

Table 4.1 Sharing Thoughts and Feelings

Skills for sharing emotions

- State your views as your own feelings and thoughts.
- Say how you are feeling or express your emotions.
- When talking about your partner, say how you feel about your partner, not just about a situation.
- Include positive feelings when you want to say something negative about something or someone.
- Keep what you want to say short and specific.
- Try not to talk for more than 30 seconds, speaking for a long time will make it hard for your partner to listen and stay focused.
- Please use tact (be kind) and think about the timing of what you want to say so it is easier for your partner to listen without getting defensive.

Skills for listening to your partner

- Show you have understood what your partner is saying by nodding, your tone of voice, facial expression and posture.
- Try to put yourself in your partner's shoes-see it from their perspective so you understand why they think and feel the way they do.
- Do not ask questions unless you need some clarification.
- Do not express your own views or opinions.
- Do not interrupt.
- Do not interpret or change the meaning of what they have said.
- Do not make judgements about what they have said.
- Do not interpret or change the meaning of their statement.

Ways to respond after your partner finishes speaking

- Summarise key thoughts, feelings, conflicts and desires.
- Check with them if you have understood what they said.

(Adapted from Baucom et al., 2019)

to think about the different demands on their relationship. They agreed the following strategies to address their concerns:

- Diaz would have a Portuguese-style breakfast with the children once a week with Fleur's support in managing them;
- They resumed date nights one evening a week; and
- They had a coffee evening to share thoughts and feelings.

Case Study Two

Simon (32) and his wife Baljit (31) struggled with how Simon's anxiety got in the way of him supporting Baljit when they were with Simon's family. Simon had a brain injury when he was 25 years old. He was on the way to work when he was hit by a car. This left him with a moderate brain injury, resulting in challenges with planning, memory, anxiety, and low self-esteem. He and Baljit had been together for two years and were living in the same home. Baljit was the first non-White person in Simon's family, which she described as 'right-winged English'. Baljit reported that they often made inappropriate comments on the family WhatsApp group about COVID, Brexit, and Black Lives Matter. It is important to say that these details were not present in the referral to the neuropsychologist (NB). They were referred for couple therapy to support Simon's adjustment to living with brain injury. The couple raised the family's communication as an issue after questions were asked about the impact of their intersecting identities on their relationship. As this issue was central to their relationship survival, it could not be avoided, nor did the neuropsychologist wish to. Using the sharing thoughts and feelings guidelines, previous ways of addressing this issue were explored. Each partner was supported to understand how the issue left the other feeling. Simon was confronted with how hurt and lonely Baljit felt when racist comments were made by his family, whilst Baljit was supported to reflect on how the brain injury contributed to Simon's response.

The couple agreed the following interventions:

- Simon agreed to educate himself on White privilege, what it means, and how it impacted on his relationship with Baljit.
- Simon agreed to speak to his family about the impact of the WhatsApp message comments on his partner.
- Baljit agreed to support Simon on the mechanics of carrying out those tasks, e.g., supporting him in putting alarm prompts on his phone to speak to the family.

The couple had other challenges that were raised in therapy. Simon found himself jealous of Baljit's successful career. When explored, themes around gender, able-ness, and ethnicity emerged. Simon reflected on how hard it was to see his girlfriend do well and to have more knowledge than him. At one point in the treatment, he asked, 'Have I got White man syndrome?' In other words, is there more to this than my brain injury? As neuropsychologists, it can be easy to dismiss his reaction as low self-esteem secondary to brain injury without exploring the multi-layers that influenced his thoughts, beliefs, and ideas. For example, what role did dominant narratives in society on race, gender, and ethnicity have in those thoughts and beliefs, and were they harmful to the couple? These themes are critical to explore given the already documented disparities in health and mental health care among marginalised populations, including those with disability and their carers. The risk of not exploring these issues in our brain injury population could result in increased strain on the couple's relationship as well as increased carer burden. According to O'Keeffe et al. (2020), research exploring the impact that brain injury has on couple relationships is limited. They found that in relationships where one partner had a brain injury, there was significant disruption of psychological well-being for both partners. O'Keeffe et al. (2020) also found a destabilisation of existing relationship dynamics; however, they suggest that brain injury does not inevitably lead to separation or breakdown of relationships. Rather, it was the lack of knowledge about potential changes that negatively impacted relationships and increased levels of psychological distress. O'Keeffe et al. (2020) suggest that for some couples the support of hope, effort, and knowledge about the impact of brain injury – not just on the brain and the individual but also on the couple and the wider family – may be therapeutic.

A position paper on supporting carers of people with progressive neurological conditions notes the significant financial implications and costs related to carer support, stating 'Neurological or behavioural symptoms such as problems with speaking or memory, or changes in mood and character can be distressing for carers as they can be difficult to predict, complicate care, and affect personal relationships' (Boele et al., 2022, p. 1). Carers' support was valued at £530 million per day in the COVID-19 pandemic (or £193 billion a year), which was more than the UK's annual health spending (Boele et al., 2022). It stands to reason that carers need good support to maintain their own health so they can provide good-quality care. A breakdown of this important relationship would lead to further strain on health and social care systems. Supporting carers means providing a space where the mental health needs of partners and families of those with brain injury can be addressed. In particular, due attention must be paid to contextual factors that may contribute to further strain in the couple relationship. Below is some guidance that neuropsychologists may find useful in adapting their approach to take intersectionality into consideration.

Guidance on Navigating Intersectionality

- Neuropsychologists should ensure that the social history taken from individuals and their families is thorough. They could review literature on identities they are less familiar with and have discussions with colleagues who may have a better understanding.
- Questions to reflect on include: On what dimensions of identity do I differ from the patient (as indicated by the demographics collected)? What blind spots may I have as a result, and what do I need to do to mitigate this? How might I unintentionally oppress the patient(s) if I'm not careful? What aspects of intersectionality exist within the individual, couple, or family system I am treating? How might I unintentionally reinforce problematic power dynamics within the system? What common stereotypes exist about the patient's identity that could unconsciously influence my work with them? How comfortable/uncomfortable am I with addressing the aspects of intersectionality I have identified?
- Neuropsychologists should check for biases or stereotypes they may possess toward certain identities.
- Neuropsychologists should use formulation models that allow for the intersectionality of both the neuropsychologist and the client.
- Neuropsychologists who are further along in this journey should seek training, consultation, and supervision to think critically about their positioning and how that intersects with the patients' identities.

Further Training

Lastly, it is clearly important to acknowledge that the vast majority of clinical neuropsychologists are thoughtful clinicians who wish the best for their patients. However, it is not enough to attend an unconscious bias training, which is the statutory response to issues of diversity and inclusion. This approach runs the risk of being highly reductionist and overgeneralising due to its ethos of moving towards 'cultural competence', which assumes an all-knowing position. However, it is impossible to grasp all the details and nuances of every intersection. Another approach is for one to take the position of curiosity, which opens up dialogue, reflects, questions, and encourages continuous learning. This is the stance of cultural humility, a concept that is discussed further in Chapter 11.

Conclusion

It is common for neuropsychologists working with couples to focus on single aspects of identity. However, to address the complex needs of couples with brain injury, the socio-political environment in which lives are lived must be attended to. Research suggests that not attending to multi-aspects of identity when working therapeutically is problematic and can lead to poorer outcomes. There are approaches which lend themselves to working intersectionally, but there is still some way to go before we, as neuropsychologists, can hold a position of humility when working contextually.

References

Ahsan, S. (2020). Holding up the mirror: Deconstructing whiteness in clinical psychology. *Journal of Critical Psychology, Counselling and Psychotherapy*, *20*(3), 45–55.

Ali, S., & Lee, C. C. (2019). Using creativity to explore intersectionality in counseling. *Journal of Creativity in Mental Health*, *14*(4), 510–518. DOI: 10.1080/15401383.2019.1632767

Atkinson, D. R. (1983). Ethnic minority representation in counsellor education. *Counselor Education and Supervision*, *23*(1), 7–19. DOI: 10.1002/j.1556-6978.1983.tb00583.x.

Backhaus, S., Neumann, D., Parrot, D., Hammond, F. M., Brownson, C., & Malec, J. (2016). Examination of an intervention to enhance relationship satisfaction after brain injury: A feasibility study. *Brain Injury*, *30*(8), 975–985. DOI: 10.3109/02699052.2016.1147601.

Baucom, D. H., Epstein, N. B., LaTaillade, J. J., & Kirby, J. S. (2008). Cognitive-behavioral couple therapy. In A. S. Gurman & N. S. Jacobson (Eds.), *Clinical handbook of couple therapy* (4th ed., 31–72). Guilford.

Baucom, D. H., Fischer, M. S., Corrie, S., Worrell, M., & Boeding, S. E. (2019). *Treating relationship distress and psychopathology in couples: A cognitive-behavioural approach*. Routledge.

Boele, F., Nicklin, E., Bronsdon, S., Brooke Mawson, I., Buckle, P., Cartwright, S., ... & Wright, J. (2022). *Supporting carers of people with a progressive neurological condition*. Position Statement 1, Policy Leeds, University of Leeds. DOI: 10.48785/100/87.

Bowen, C., Palmer, S., & Yeates, G. (2018). *A relational approach to rehabilitation: Thinking about relationships after brain injury*. Routledge. (Original work published 2010).

Brah, A., & Phoenix, A. (2004). Ain't I a woman?: Revisiting Intersectionality. *Journal of International Women's Studies*, *5*(3), 75–86.

Channon, S., & Crawford, S. (2010). Mentalising and social problem-solving after brain injury. *Neuropsychological Rehabilitation*, *20*(5), 739–759. DOI: 10.1080/09602011003794583.

Doidge, N. (2008). *The brain that changes itself: Stories of personal triumph from the frontiers of brain science*. Penguin.

Eubanks, C. F., Burckell, L. A., & Goldfried, M. R. (2018). Clinical consensus strategies to repair ruptures in the therapeutic alliance. *Journal of Psychotherapy Integration*, *28*(1), 60–76. DOI: 10.1037/int0000097.

Godwin, E. E., Kreutzer, J. S., Arango-Lasprilla, J. C., & Lehan, T. J. (2011). Marriage after brain injury: Review, analysis, and research recommendations. *Journal of Head Trauma Rehabilitation*, *26*(1), 43–55. DOI: 10.1097/HTR.0b013e3182048f54.

Hammond, F. M., Sevigny, M., Backhaus, S., Neumann, D., Corrigan, J. D., Charles, S. K., & Gazett, H. (2021). Marital Stability Over 10 Years Following Traumatic Brain Injury, *Journal of Head Trauma Rehabilitation*, *36*(4) , 199–208.

Kim, E., & Kang, M. (2018). The effects of client–counselor racial matching on therapeutic outcome. *Asia Pacific Educ. Rev.*, *19*, 103–110. DOI: 10.1007/s12564-018-9518-9

Klonoff, P. S. (2014). *Psychotherapy for families after brain injury*. Springer Science & Business.

Lieberman, M. D. (2007). Social cognitive neuroscience: A review of core processes. *Annual Review of Psychology*, *58*, 259–289. DOI: 10.1146/annurev.psych.58.110405.085654.

O'Keeffe, F., Dunne, J., Nolan, M., Cogley, C., & Davenport, J. (2020). 'The things that people can't see': The impact of TBI on relationships: An interpretative phenomenological analysis. *Brain Injury*, *34*(4), 496–507. DOI: 10.1080/02699052.2020.1725641

Ownsworth, T. (2014). *Self-identity after brain injury*. Psychology Press.

PettyJohn, M. E., Tseng, C. F., & Blow, A. J. (2020). Therapeutic utility of discussing therapist/client intersectionality in treatment: When and how?. *Family Process*, *59*(2), 313–327. DOI: 10.1111/famp.12471.

Review of *Escape from Babel: Toward a unifying language for psychotherapy practice* by Miller, S. D., Duncan, B. L., & Hubble, M. A. (1997). *Adolescence*, *32*(125), 247.

Stiekema, A. P. M., Resch, C., Donkervoort, M., Jansen, N., Jurrius, K. H. M., Zadoks, J. M., & van Heugten, C. M. (2020). Case management after acquired brain injury compared to care as usual: Study protocol for a 2-year pragmatic randomized controlled superiority trial with two parallel groups. *Trials*, *21*(928), 1–16. DOI: 10.1186/s13063-020-04804-2.

Stuart, R. B. (1969). Operant-interpersonal treatment for marital discord. *Journal of Consulting and Clinical Psychology*, *33*(6), 675–682. DOI: 10.1037/h0028475.

Thibaut, J. W., & Kelley, H. H. (1959). *The social psychology of groups*. Wiley Publications.

5 Hidden Social Inequalities in Paediatric Neurorehabilitation

Jenny Jim, Gemma Costello, Valéria Lowing, Steve Nash, Chezelle Scholes and Alison Perkins

Introduction

Acquired brain injury (ABI) is the leading cause of disability in childhood (Forsyth & Kirkham, 2012). The National Institute for Health and Care Excellence (NICE) estimates that almost 40,000 brain injuries in children under 16 years present to accident and emergency departments each year in England (NICE, 2014). Most of these children will have a traumatic brain injury (such as those resulting from road traffic accidents, assaults, falls, etc.). In addition, hundreds of children will acquire a brain injury through non-traumatic means (such as through stroke, brain tumour, or infection, e.g., meningitis or encephalitis). These injuries can vary from mild to severe. Whilst a spectrum of severity exists, life-changing impacts can occur at any level.

Children, young people, and families (CYPF) with ABI face hidden social, physical, emotional, cognitive, and spiritual/identity impacts (see Jim & Norton, 2015), which are often represented using the metaphor of an iceberg. Many will show excellent visible recovery, but a myriad of ABI impacts remains invisible. This may include: difficulties with concentration, memory, processing, planning, organisation, impulsivity, social competency, sleep, emotional lability, irritability, motor-coordination, emotional well-being, trauma, and multiple types of fatigue as well as visual-perceptual difficulties, sensory difficulties, chronic pain, headaches, and other health problems.

Having an ABI can additionally place the CYPF in a vicious cycle with social adversities, whereby risks to future quality of life have the potential to grow exponentially. For the general population, the interaction of adverse childhood events (ACEs) on health, social, and mental health outcomes is becoming increasingly recognised (Anda et al., 2010). We would like to propose the idea of balancing the picture with a focus on adverse social-political elements (ASPs) that underlie social inequality within the systems/contexts that specifically negatively affect CYPF with ABI.

'Social inequality' conceptualises the uneven distribution of goods (e.g., wealth, income, education, employment, access to health or social care) and burdens (e.g., poor physical or mental health, poverty,

DOI: 10.4324/9781003309819-7

marginalisation, criminality) between societal groups (often categorised by gender, ethnicity, age, the presence of disabilities, or parental status).

We would like to demonstrate our process and outcomes of personal and professional reflection that have brought us to a sense of what we need to take more action on. By highlighting and mitigating against avoidable ASPs, we can increase the chances that our CYPF can truly live with their ABI.

We invite you on our journey, hoping it may give ideas to you in your context. We take a non-expert approach, based on a narrative position, seeking multiplicity of views that we see as equally valid. This is simply the way that one team has tried to authentically engage in the process and embrace uncomfortable 'truths' that may emerge from it. We all accept that our clinical space is likely to provide a stage for the re-enactment of our own social-political norms and inequities.

Author Context

The authors of this chapter are members of the Psychosocial Service at The Children's Trust. The Children's Trust is a charity that is commissioned by NHS England to provide national specialist inpatient neurorehabilitation to children, young people, and families with ABI. Residential rehabilitation offers a full range of therapies and education to support them in meeting their goals for meaningful participation.

Our service provides social work, music therapy, youth work, clinical psychology, educational psychology, and neuropsychology. The team have extensive experience in working with the inpatient residential context and community settings across the local authority, schools, health and mental health. We work as part of a wider interdisciplinary team, providing inpatient and community-focused rehabilitation to children, young people, and their families.

Our service aims to provide intensive support to respond to needs around well-being, identity, models of trauma-informed care, psychoeducation, systemic support, neuropsychological assessment, and rehabilitation, whilst also connecting families to systems within the community that can take a longer-term role in supporting their needs.

Overview

ASPs come in many forms, with roots in societal, cultural, and political beliefs that have the power to define what is seen, what is recognised, and what is then responded to – thereby enshrining these in the way our services work (or don't work), and whose needs are prioritised and why. Our institutions, which are meant to serve the diversities of our population, can unintentionally become the material manifestation of common, uninformed, or prejudicial beliefs.

For instance, for CYPF with ABI, a couple of key myths within society and culture are that children 'bounce back' due to plasticity and that this population is very small. This leads to inaction with regards to changes to our current provisions, as they are not seen to be needed. There is an under-recognition of and under-provision (even when acknowledged) for the cumulative risk that follows childhood brain injury, which sees the increased likelihood of exploitation, academic and vocational under-achievement, and contact with criminal justice system (Williams, 2012).

Developing a comprehensive and authentic understanding of the roots to these issues is crucial to inform effective, sustainable responses. Currently, the risks and resiliencies within our systems/service remain unexamined to the degree that CYPF affected by ABI deserve.

Our children do not 'bounce back' in the way society may believe (see long-term studies by Anderson et al., 2005). We are also facing a 'hidden epidemic' on a global level (All-Party Parliamentary Group on ABI, 2018). The prevalence of traumatic brain injury alone (which excludes brain injuries such as those sustained via brain infections, tumours, and bleeds) in children and young people (CYP) is estimated to be as high as almost 32%. This figure dwarfs that for CYP with ASD, ADHD, LD, and dyslexia put together, which is 24% in total (NASEN and the Child Brain Injury Trust, 2018).

Despite this, it is an optimistic time for those committed to improving the lives of CYPF with ABI. Collective efforts from the field are creating opportunities for greater visibility of myriad factors that impact on the rights of CYPF with ABI. Momentum is gaining following the All-Party Parliamentary Group on Acquired Brain Injury's (APPG) 'Time for Change' recommendations on ABI (2018). The APPG has representation across government departments, including Education, Health and Social Care, Work and Pensions, Digital Culture Media and Sport, and the Ministry of Justice, which aimed to unite a strategy across departments to drive change for brain injury survivors.

A green light has been given by the government to implement a cross-departmental strategy for ABI. This collaborative effort from service users, providers, supporters, and MPs brings an opportunity for powerful advocacy and culminates in a need to no longer ignore the inequalities people affected by ABI face. An analogous stepwise change in recognising the need for more fully networked understandings and actions for ABI can be seen in historical philosophies of the brain, whereby localisation theories were eventually replaced by connectionist models.

Lifespan Risk and Resiliency Factors Should Not be Ignored

Whilst we very much welcome the proposed cross-departmental nature of the new strategy, this should not take precedence over a lifespan risk and resiliency approach. This is crucial for meeting the needs of CYPF with ABI. In our view, important ministers are often unseen or might be overlooked as key stakeholders in current systems, such as those that address the rights of women (including addressing gender-based violence and domestic abuse); access to high-quality maternity, perinatal, post-natal care, and early years' services (such as the Minister for Women and Equalities and the Minister for Patient Safety and Primary Care); and those that engage fathers and other guardians.

Supporting primary caregivers allows them to give the care and nurturance to their children for the best neuroadvantages in life. Support may include equality in pay for women so that they can have greater opportunities to provide materially and emotionally for their children. This can result in changing discourses on the value of caregiving, understanding the links between secure attachment with brain development and longer-term outcomes, which all increase the chances that we do not as a society disadvantage the neurological bedrock of the children of parents/ caregivers who may already be navigating layers of social adversity.

Psychosocial factors such as positive parental involvement, emotional wellbeing, and access to material and social resources are key in long-term outcomes for CYPF with ABI (Yeates et al., 2010). We need to create the conditions whereby the presence of these positive factors is not dependent on existing privileges and power.

Inequalities We Witness and Owning Our Involvement in Perpetuating Inequality

We see multiple inequalities throughout the system and our practice. On a human level we witness CYPF struggle to have a voice that is listened to and understood. Key questions in our minds are: How can we empower all families, not just those that have the privileges to be able to attend and be attended to in specialist services, such as White, middle-class families? What would a non-ableist and non-Western approach to rehabilitation look like? How do we replicate existing social stigmas/inequalities/privileges? Who do our structures and processes favour? Who is not seen or excluded? What are the unintended consequences of our systems, such as reinforcing traditional gender roles or problematising non-Western cultural beliefs/values/behaviours?

Changes are required so that the complexity of need is reflected with appropriate and timely normalised provision, e.g., service for CYPF to adjust and adapt to life following a significant physical and psychological trauma. As it stands today, a young person who sustains a significant brain injury following an attempt on their life due to challenges with their mental health has a fragmented pathway to longer-term support. They find themselves in a vicious circle, whereby they are even less able to advocate their needs, be actively listened to, and then to access services on offer. They often fall between services, which exist with a lack of empirically informed proactive support, or risk entering a system that pathologises an appropriate emotional response to trauma.

Inequalities over access to valued activities, such as satisfying higher education and employment (Gormley et al., 2019; Willmott et al., 2014) or social and physical leisure activities (Katz-Leurer et al., 2010; Keetley et al., 2021), are magnified for CYP with ABI. This results in much greater social disablement than would be indicated by need. We must be transparent that drivers for neurorehabilitation are a product of certain parts of our society, as discussed in Chapter 1, and they reflect the beliefs that these people hold. Our context is an ever-changing political landscape, which at this stage brings us unprecedented opportunity for positive change.

Whilst listing the above important factors, we feel the discomfort in our inherent complicity with these. We must own these feelings and ask ourselves: What can you/we do more of? What are you/we waiting for? What changes have you/we driven forward, and which ones get left on the back burner? Is 'the system' the real block to changing? Who is understood by the system? Or is the way you/we do or do not mobilise together to find a new way of working a hindrance?

We realise that as a team we need to not only to focus on the 'top-down' influences but also the responsibilities we have with the use of our power in a 'bottom-up' direction. The team saw the invitation to contribute a chapter to this book as a welcome invitation to learn about ourselves.

The Unsaid or Unheeded Structural Inequalities that Put CYP at Elevated Risk of ABI

Childhood ABI does not operate within an equal opportunities' basis – this is especially so for traumatic brain injury (TBI), whereby ASPs, such as poverty, financial disadvantage, less-enriched social environments, and intergenerational factors (social, psychological, and genetic), combine to elevate the risk of acquiring an injury. An example of this is how some of the above factors may lead to an elevated risk of receiving a diagnosis of ADHD, which increases the risk of a TBI by virtue of less aversion to risk, inadequate supervision, and increased impulsivity, leading to behaviours that carry greater likelihood of injury. There may be less obvious pathways. For example, children who sustain developmental trauma through early adverse life events may develop survival responses, such as hyperarousal, self-reliance, dissociation, and learnt helplessness (van der Kolk, 2005). As these children mature, these strategies can underpin personal beliefs, social network selection, and coping strategies (Lyons et al., 2020; Raby & Jones, 2016) that increase the risk of an ABI through increased risk-taking (Odacı & Çelik, 2020), substance abuse, or suicidal behaviour (Dye, 2018; Miller et al., 2013).

Neurodevelopmental risk (e.g., a diagnosis of ASD) may even combine with the scenario above, leading to uncertainty as to who is best placed to respond to their needs. This demonstrates the accumulation of adversity across time, which is likely to exponentially impact trajectories of recovery.

It is well known that Black and ethnic minority groups are over-represented within the population of CYP in custody. Of all CYP remanded into custody in England and Wales between March 2019 and March 2020, 43% were of White ethnicity, 35% were Black, 14% were mixed, and 9% were of Asian or other type of ethnicity (Youth Justice Board & Ministry of Justice, 2021). Evidence tracking the long-term trajectories of CYP with ABI reveals that this group, too, is over-represented. Williams (2012) found that 60% of CYP in custody have experienced a TBI, in line with international findings. This tells us that we need to change our services.

Though TBI is the leading cause of ABI in CYP, we cannot ignore the disadvantages experienced by those living with the sequelae of brain tumours, strokes, infections, and hypoxic events. These groups are often recognised within health systems but may fail to come to the attention of education, care, mental health, and other community-based provision. The nature of how these injuries are acquired brings a risk of diagnostic over-shadowing.

Neuropsychological evidence tells us that CYP require access to long-term follow up, which challenges our current models of working. Awareness of ABI is growing, and the hope is that political, commissioning, and service leaders can move beyond awareness to action, developing pathways and provision that meet CYPF needs.

It could be argued that the socio-political conditions are more favourable at this time for a widespread acceptance of neurodiversity. Since The Autism Act (2009), there have been strategic and structural changes across health, social, and education services with everyday awareness and acceptance. It is our hope that the conceptual groundwork has been laid for ABI with an agreed cross-departmental, all-party parliamentary strategy that seeks to align the evidence base with service delivery.

There is also a workforce issue, in that training programmes sponsored by the Department of Health and Social Care (e.g., clinical psychology, social work, and allied health professionals) and the Department for Education (e.g., teacher training and educational psychology) give little priority to a holistic understanding of brain development, the primary and secondary impacts of brain injury, and the importance of being responsive to emerging needs across the lifespan.

Team Exercise 1: Mapping Our View of ASPs in Paediatric Neurorehabilitation

We used the systems from the ecological systems model (Bronfenbrenner, 1979) to reflect as a team about ASPs. These were explored in the context of those we were consciously aware of and gave voice to unsaid

What we know

Intrapersonal
social inequalities increasing risk of ABI; sex differences; ACEs, Neurodiversity; caregiving experiences affect neurodevelopment; brain behaviour links; typical development trajectories may be altered; CYP's voice is paramount.

Interpersonal
Family functioning is crucial; dynamic interplay between resources and lived experience; promotion of 'good enough' caregiving; different norms within cultures; perceptions of disability; ambiguous loss, trauma responses, loss of peer relationships; peer acceptance; frameworks of meaning; diversity of narratives of the future; contextual safeguarding risks.

Organisational
Inequity of access/service; lack of services; unresponsive/overwhelmed systems; postcode lottery; cumulative disadvantage; insufficient housing stock; homeowner status; lack of confidence/ competence re. ABI; diagnostic overshadowing; physical and mental health services lack integration; invisibility/ lack of awareness; myths re. ABI.

Community
lack of awareness of ABI; lack of ownership; poor incidence reporting and monitoring; passive system; reliance on pockets of best practice; reliance on goodwill; limited access to the rehab code; inequity amongst types of ABI; different recognition of psychosocial need.

Society
lack of awareness/responsibility of ABI; implicit dualism- lack of integration of mind and body; mindset issue; spiritual/identity/cultural influences not taken into account; disability is a societal construct; psychosocial protection and risk factors; no ABI strategy/pathways - socio-political inequity.

What we want to do more of

Intrapersonal
understanding neuro-disadvantage; exploring CYP lived experience more deeply; respect individual impacts of social inequality; connecting identity and rehab, telling more empowering stories; increasing accessibility and participation; increasing acceptance and value within society.

Interpersonal
allowing subjugated stories to be told, post-traumatic growth; promoting mastery, understanding intersectionality, active mitigation against contextual safeguarding risks; whole family involvement; involvement of fathers.

Organisational
identifying pockets of good practice/agents of change; investing in /influencing organisational vision/change; improving our evidence and research; utilising research to design services; embedding theory practice links; responding to and influencing the commissioning landscape.

Community
operationalising what effective system looks like; utilising family/community support.

Society
Greater understanding of how ABI is viewed in different cultures; operationalising collectivist oriented and/ or non-ableist rehab; greater awareness of how society limits those living with ABI; creating attitude change; labelling inherent belief systems that are embedded in our services; deconstructing disability; moving to action re. ACEs, socialGRACES; what impact there may be of a strategy.

(centre axis label: ASPs, Social GRACES, Lifespan approach, ACEs, construct of disability; family life cycles)

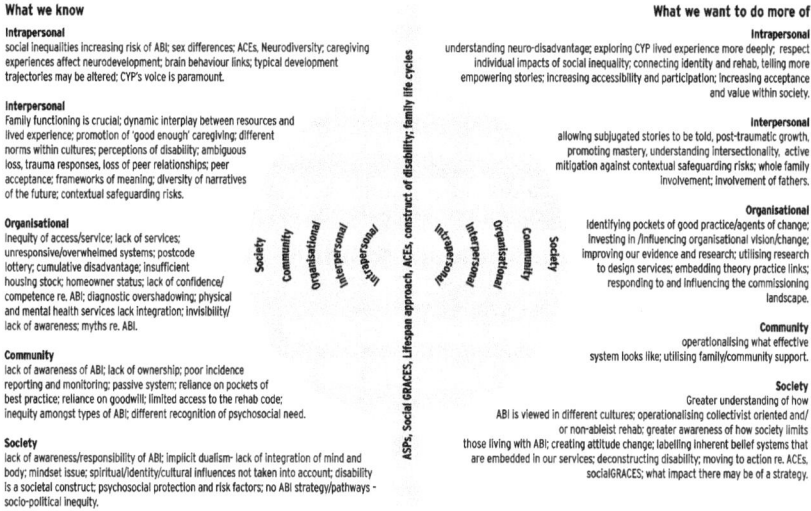

Figure 5.1 Team Awareness of Social Inequalities and Other Key Factors in Pae-diatric Neurorehabilitation

or previously unknown to us factors that might influence CYPF out-comes and lived experience. We aimed to bring to our own awareness the interacting factors that we felt were consciously 'known' and to raise questions of what we needed to know more about or do more about. We started with mentalising the CYP's experience, then we explored wider circles around the CYP, such as family, peers, community, and society.

This is presented in Figure 5.1 below, with the left-hand side of the image depicting our conscious awareness and the right-hand side depicting what we need to learn more about. The figure presents our baseline understand-ing of ecosystemic factors at play within neurorehabilitation. We noticed how much inequity existed and how much we still need to action.

Conversations: Exploring Narratives of CYPF's Lived Experience

It was of paramount importance that CYPF were able to share their per-spectives and lived experience. We provided space for them to tell the stories they felt able to share with a clinician that they knew well. Our role was to listen to the dominant narratives whilst also listening for any unsaid or subjugated narratives that may have been too threatening to express.

We present synopses of five narratives from CYPF, which include three CYP and two now adults who experienced childhood ABI and were keen to speak with us.

Charlotte (25 years old) *'Brain injury behind the scenes'*

Charlotte is from a White British background, and she sustained a severe brain injury at the age of 11 years on a family holiday. She had a ruptured arteriovenous malformation and aneurysm.

Whilst she made a very good recovery, with no outward signs of having experienced an ABI, she spoke about lasting impacts upon making and maintaining friendships and securing suitable employment. In order to find employment in her chosen vocation, she made the decision to not disclose her health history because she feared she would be discriminated against and judged by her ABI and not her skills. We noticed the strong influence of social stigma as well as the interaction of hiding her ABI and therefore not being able to seek reasonable adaptations when fulfilling her role.

Charlotte believed that sharing the fact that she had an ABI would risk losing her income, leading to a decline in her mental health. We noticed that Charlotte was in a cycle of cumulative disadvantage, whereby factors such as real and perceived stigma ended up restricting her opportunities and earning potential. Charlotte has great strengths in employing coping strategies, e.g., pacing to manage her fatigue. Charlotte also shared that she felt others had made decisions for her, which they deemed to be in her best interests, and this had not been welcomed. Charlotte advocated for shared decision-making and being supported for advocating her needs.

Lorenzzo (14 years old) *'Having an ABI brings limitations but should not stop you'*

Lorenzzo is a friendly young person who describes himself as having a good sense of humour and enjoys being connected with others and engaging in social activities. His interests extend to online computer games, football, cycling, spending time with animals, nature, and horse riding. He is originally from Brazil and moved to the UK in 2020. He is an only child and lives at home with his parents. He describes his ethnicity as Brazilian and Italian.

Lorenzzo was hit by a car while cycling and sustained a severe ABI with bilateral haemorrhages, cerebral oedema, and acute axonal injury. He also sustained several physical injuries. Lorenzzo experiences a range of needs across physical, communication, and cognitive domains. Lorenzzo communicates verbally primarily in Portuguese.

Independence was a recurring theme of importance to Lorenzzo and underpinned much of his narrative. Lorenzzo spoke of wanting to go out on his own and how his parents did not currently allow this. He recognises that adults worry about his safety and therefore aim to keep him safe. While Lorenzzo enjoys being at home and gaming, he feels being restricted in his movements 'only makes things worse'. Lorenzzo is gaining independence through a three-days-a-week support worker provided by

Children's Social Care in his local area and hopes 'in the future maybe' he will work towards going out on his own.

Lorenzzo shared previous experiences of bullying when at school in Brazil and, whilst awaiting a new school in the UK, he shared concerns that 'going to school is harder now' and expressed feeling 'worried about going to a new school' due to concerns about making friends as well as worries of being 'treated like a baby'. Lorenzzo does not see his language as a barrier to social equality as he is learning English, but he recognises that since his ABI it 'can be a problem when you don't have access to the right adaptations or help'.

Lorenzzo uses online platforms to meet, make, and maintain social relationships to reduce social isolation. We know that seeking relationships online can present a risk of abuse and exploitation. Vulnerability to online risks may increase, particularly while he is limited in opportunities to access a peer group via education or within community spaces.

Lorenzzo experiences online bullying when interacting with others – 'People have made fun of me sometimes when I'm playing online' – and attributes this to his changed voice tone and speed. Our understating is that Lorenzzo seeks comfort in interactions that allow him to be accepted by his peers. The online world allows him to be himself for more of the time, participating just like everybody else. He remains aware of others' potential negative perceptions of difference.

Lorenzzo had three main messages to share: to other young people with an ABI – 'Never give up'; to his peers – 'Don't make fun of anyone. You don't know what is going on for them'; and to professionals and adults – 'Don't think that a young person with an ABI is not capable. They are still capable of achieving things'.

Afiya (15 years old) and Her Mother *'Supporting CYPF with awareness and openness'*

Afiya is a young person of Jamaican and Ugandan descent. She felt a strong connection to family, speaking openly, building relationships with others, the importance of eating and enjoying food together, and the belief that family always comes first.

Afiya sustained a traumatic brain injury following an accident where she was hit by a car at a pedestrian crossing. She sustained a severe ABI. Afiya's primary areas of need were in relation to cognitive communication, some residual weakness on her right side, cognitive needs, and understandable emotional trauma.

During rehabilitation Afiya was able to name what she perceived to be a system that was not reflective of her race or cultural values. Afiya would organise her day to spend time with her family, which she was able to identify as going against some of the expectations of a typical neurorehabilitation day. This in turn led to tensions with staff, who misinterpreted a cultural and values-based decision to be with family as stepping outside of the rules or expectations for the service. Afiya and her family were able to name this. They spoke about their culture, their race, and how it felt to be a minoritised ethnic group in a predominantly White environment, and they challenged the team to reflect on positions of privilege and bias in models of service delivery and expectations.

Afiya shared that on her return to school she 'just wanted to feel like everybody else'. Above all, her priority was to be accepted by her peers and 'fit in'. This was the driving force behind her wishes to return to school with things as 'normal' as they could be. This appeared to be centred around Afiya's awareness that her ABI could bring about judgements or stigma from peers who perceived her to be 'different'. It is only now, over time, that Afiya has shared that whilst 'I want to feel like everyone else, I do realise that I need support'. This concept reinforces the need for dynamic and responsive systems that can respond to emerging needs of CYPF following ABI.

Afiya also identified that on her return to school, it was challenging when teachers tried to encourage her to have relationships with peers with 'additional needs'. She felt the pressure to conform to a new group, one that was determined by their similar needs rather than shared interests. She felt that pressure from teachers and was able to articulate: 'Just because I have needs, it doesn't mean I have to make friends with other people who do too'. This was a powerful narrative and one where Afiya is both able to acknowledge her needs post-ABI and, crucially, separate them from her identity and how she sees herself as a peer to her friends.

Afiya was able to identify the challenges that teachers and other professionals face in understanding ABI. She and her mother referred to this as 'Some people just don't understand, and they make mistakes, but they need to understand if they are to support everyone'. This brings an interesting challenge to the education, health, and care professions, where there is a need for greater awareness of the sequelae of ABI and what CYPF want from the services that might support them. Crucially, Afiya shared narratives of hope, 'I don't think of the worst, I think of the best. I am still the same old Afiya. It's just the little things that have changed'.

Afiya's mother reflected upon how she felt staff avoided speaking with her about issues or concerns, instead reporting them to others, despite their everyday conversations. She felt like 'they were almost scared to speak to me, making me feel like quite a scary person'. This was explored in the context of narratives that exist of Black women and/or the avoidance of potential conflict or difficult conversations.

Richard (20 years old) *'Paramount support, resilience, and continuity of identity and goals'*

Richard is from a White British background, and he sustained a brain injury at the age of 15. He had a presumed idiopathic encephalitis. Richard met each of his rehabilitation goals whilst on placement and successfully transitioned back to his community without the need for additional support from children's social care.

When asked to reflect on his current circumstances, Richard felt no particular disadvantages due to his health history. He has continued to meet his developmental milestones educationally and in areas of employment due to his own perseverance and the holistic support of his parents. His parents understood that his stage of development required skilled adaptation to new environments, skills, and practices depending on the occupational and education choices which he would make. He was supported through work experience to develop skills and interests in childcare, which have enabled him to progress both vocationally and educationally within a supportive work and learning environment.

Living at home and within the continuum of past and present loving parental care enables Richard to navigate his life with confidence and grow in the directions he wisely chooses to take. Through their carefulness, his parents enable their son's engagement with life experiences which support him to reach his potential. Richard maintains his connections with The Children's Trust through participation events, which enable him to have a say in aspects of the organisation and its future, and he has expressed how much this adds to his sense of belonging and community.

Yuusuf (14 years old) and His Family *'Faith, family, love, and unconditional acceptance'*

Yuusuf is a young man who is very loved by his parents and seven siblings. Yuusuf's family are from Somalia, and their faith is Islam.

Yusuf sustained a traumatic brain injury when he was hit by a car. Yuusuf sustained a severe ABI and was in disorder of consciousness prior to commencing neurorehabilitation.

Yuusuf completed his neurorehabilitation two years ago. To date he remains in residential care due to overcrowding in the family property and a lack of housing available for him to discharge to. He expressed both sadness and anger when signing and using his AAC at the situation he finds himself in. He wishes to return to live at home. He values his regular visits to the centre and his weekly trips to home, but they also make him sad, as they bring awareness of the barriers he faces that are beyond his and the family's control.

Yuusuf has recently learnt more about his ABI, and his family have shared their understanding of his journey through their faith. They have been able to comfort Yuusuf and share messages of love and unconditional acceptance as well as, most importantly, how their faith brings understanding to his lived experience. They have shared how Yuusuf's path was set out when his sex was determined in utero, and this was his and theirs to tread together. They reinforce narratives of strength and faith, and they are so proud of him for who he is. Whilst Yuusuf is always encouraged and his many steps in recovery are celebrated, the family reinforce a message about the present and valuing him for all that he is, not what his next steps in rehabilitation might be – a lesson for us all to reflect on in sitting with the here and now.

In Yuusuf's case, the lack of responsive systems brings challenges, both from a perspective of barriers to communication that the family may face but also in the notion that sometimes only the loudest and most powerful voices can challenge social injustice. The inequities in the system present cumulative barriers for this young man to return to the loving care of his family, and they demonstrate the imbalance of power in a system that will continue to pay for costly residential care, yet will not explore other favourable, equally costly solutions that might see a young person reunited with their family.

Team Exercise 2: Mapping Lived Experience of CYPF

Team members recounted the conversations they had with the CYPF to the team, and we produced Figure 5.2, a representation of how CYPF experience the world around them post-injury.

Team Exercise 3: Understanding What We Respond To and What We Need to Do More Of

We sought to amalgamate the learning we had made across our process and felt it best captured as an iceberg. Figure 5.3 is a representation of ASPs and other factors that, as a professional system, we respond to, we

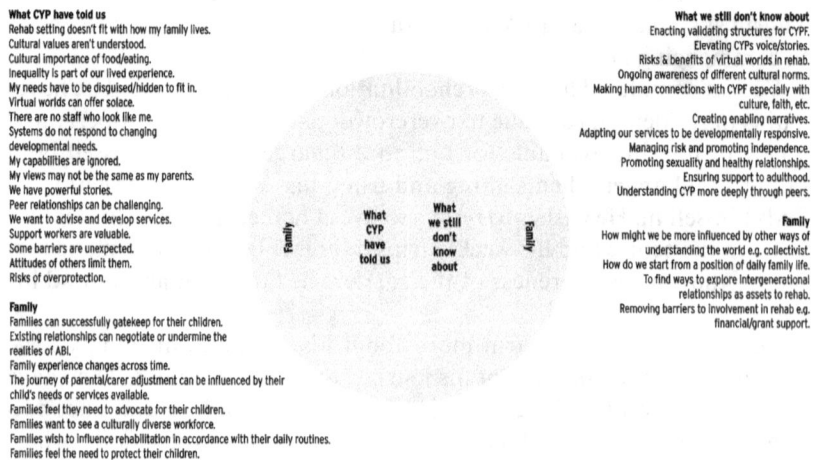

What CYP have told us
Rehab setting doesn't fit with how my family lives.
Cultural values aren't understood.
Cultural importance of food/eating.
Inequality is part of our lived experience.
My needs have to be disguised/hidden to fit in.
Virtual worlds can offer solace.
There are no staff who look like me.
Systems do not respond to changing developmental needs.
My capabilities are ignored.
My views may not be the same as my parents.
We have powerful stories.
Peer relationships can be challenging.
We want to advise and develop services.
Support workers are valuable.
Some barriers are unexpected.
Attitudes of others limit them.
Risks of overprotection.

Family
Families can successfully gatekeep for their children.
Existing relationships can negotiate or undermine the realities of ABI.
Family experience changes across time.
The journey of parental/carer adjustment can be influenced by their child's needs or services available.
Families feel they need to advocate for their children.
Families want to see a culturally diverse workforce.
Families wish to influence rehabilitation in accordance with their daily routines.
Families feel the need to protect their children.

What we still don't know about
Enacting validating structures for CYPF.
Elevating CYPs voice/stories.
Risks & benefits of virtual worlds in rehab.
Ongoing awareness of different cultural norms.
Making human connections with CYPF especially with culture, faith, etc.
Creating enabling narratives.
Adapting our services to be developmentally responsive.
Managing risk and promoting independence.
Promoting sexuality and healthy relationships.
Ensuring support to adulthood.
Understanding CYP more deeply through peers.

Family
How might we be more influenced by other ways of understanding the world e.g. collectivist.
How do we start from a position of daily family life.
To find ways to explore intergenerational relationships as assets to rehab.
Removing barriers to involvement in rehab e.g. financial/grant support.

Family | What CYP have told us | What we still don't know about | Family

Figure 5.2 Learning from CYPF's Experience

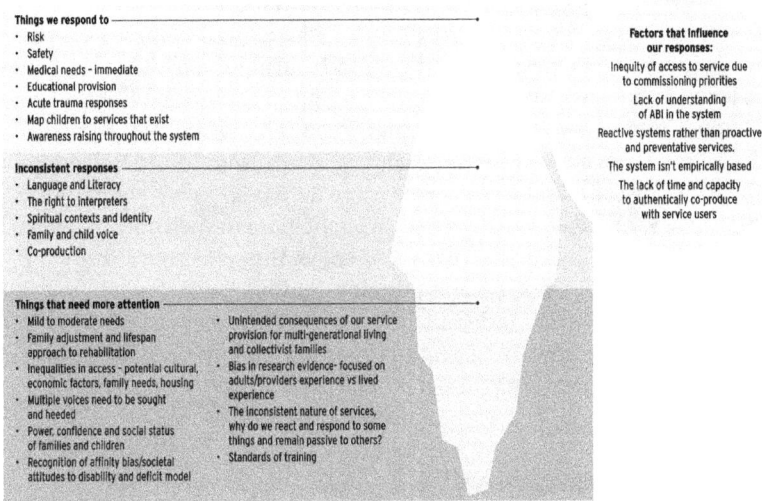

Things we respond to
- Risk
- Safety
- Medical needs – immediate
- Educational provision
- Acute trauma responses
- Map children to services that exist
- Awareness raising throughout the system

Inconsistent responses
- Language and Literacy
- The right to interpreters
- Spiritual contexts and identity
- Family and child voice
- Co-production

Things that need more attention
- Mild to moderate needs
- Family adjustment and lifespan approach to rehabilitation
- Inequalities in access – potential cultural, economic factors, family needs, housing
- Multiple voices need to be sought and heeded
- Power, confidence and social status of families and children
- Recognition of affinity bias/societal attitudes to disability and deficit model
- Unintended consequences of our service provision for multi-generational living and collectivist families
- Bias in research evidence- focused on adults/providers experience vs lived experience
- The inconsistent nature of services, why do we reect and respond to some things and remain passive to others?
- Standards of training

Factors that influence our responses:
Inequity of access to service due to commissioning priorities
Lack of understanding of ABI in the system
Reactive systems rather than proactive and preventative services.
The system isn't empirically based
The lack of time and capacity to authentically co-produce with service users

Figure 5.3 Our Current Understanding of How We Respond (or Not) to ASPs and Other Factors by Existing System

respond inconsistently to, and deserve more attention. Surrounding the iceberg are factors that influence our patterns of responding.

Mitigating Against ASPs and Ideas for Inclusive Paediatric Neurorehabilitation

We could see a range of social inequalities that resulted from ASPs. We saw that whilst we do respond to many, such as when CYPF present with risk or the need to return to education, there is a need to help existing services see how they can meet the needs of a CYF with an ABI through their existing pathways and raising awareness across the system. We also recognise that we provide highly bespoke rehabilitation programmes that focus on meaningful participation.

As a team we need to show greater consistency in our responses:

- Providing access to interpreters as well as translated, easy read, and recorded materials;
- Maintaining an open, curious, and non-judgemental approach to how care is received and utilised by CYPF when it differs from the majority of CYPF accessing services;
- Further embedding our SPECS framework across the organisation and network, which explicitly asks about spiritual contexts and identity;

- Interrupting biases through workforce recruitment and retention as well as promoting diverse voices and psychological safety;
- Creating environments that promote creativity, compassion, and inclusion, where we value speaking up and sharing diverse identities while role modelling inclusive behaviours. This might include non-ableist, collectivist, and non-Western ideals that empower and enable CYP;
- Investing the time and capacity on true co-production to look at how meetings are run and what services are delivered as well as exploring bias in who engages in or is asked to participate in such conversations;
- Challenging stigmatising views and societal norms that limit CYP's potential and promoting empowering and adequate independence/connectedness as desired; and
- Acknowledging how we use our own power and influence on systems outside of our own, e.g., housing or care packages vs. the cost of residential care.

How might we influence change?

- By forming robust global networks;
- Increasing our commitment to campaigns and national consultation, e.g., APPG, N-ABLES, NICE guidance development;
- Articulating when CAMHS or other paediatric/third-sector services might be able to meet CYPF needs post ABI;
- Reviewing our organisational policies to ensure equity of access;
- Looking actively for gaps in service provision, whilst also educating/bringing awareness of inequity to the attention of commissioners;
- Promoting our own reflexivity and that of others;
- Maintaining a position of and commitment to shared discovery and self-reflection, where our key assumption is that there will always be factors that are not currently in our awareness;
- Ensuring that research ideally informs the basis for national policy and service structures, and challenging ourselves to address bias in what is researched and who participates because, crucially, what is represented in research is what is likely to be replicated in service delivery;
- Supporting workforce readiness by promoting the need for training programmes to cover theories of brain development and holistic neurorehabilitation;
- Promoting awareness of a lifespan approach to ABI; empowering the everyday person to understand the inherent importance of opportunities for healthy relationships; and challenging ASPs in our environment as they create risks to the rights for healthy neuropsychological development;
- Celebrating and learning from services and CYPF experiences of success (according to what is important for them) enabled by their different systems;

- Developing an explicit understanding that our well-being and the presence of ASPs are connected to wider socio-political decisions; and
- Promoting subjugated narratives of ABI and adjustment.

Evaluation

As a team, the process has been invaluable in keeping conversations going about ASPs and our responsibilities in meeting the holistic needs of our CYPF with ABI.

We acknowledge the limitations of our process, which is not embedded in rigour but sits within the context of reflective practice and practice-based evidence.

We also reflected on sources of bias in our process and focus. This will have affected which CYPF's stories were elevated, what clinician chose to follow-up in conversations, and what the team deemed to be important to write about in this chapter. In addition, we wondered about different ways of engagement and the remaining silent voices.

Some team members noticed that no credence was given to obvious inequalities that are inherent in the development and applicability of neuropsychology tests to wider populations. We recognise the disadvantage this may confer on an everyday basis when results are written up in reports that mask this bias effectively with statistics that purport to represent universal 'norms' and 'base rates'.

We acknowledge the potential for bias and privilege within the system and that there may be dynamics that allow families to feel that the ABI may not have had the same level of impact as it did for others. We need to better understand the protective factors and buffers to the disadvantages of ABI. Our focus in this chapter, on the adverse socio-political elements, may mean that we have not have fully acknowledged the privileges that families experience in health systems, and this may be an area for further research.

Some team members also realised the lack of reflection on our own personal biases and why these did not come through in the conversation we had as a team. Are we also still hiding these from ourselves? Are we ready, as a neurorehabilitation service and society, for ASP dialogue and making the required changes?

Finally, we also noticed a bias in not acknowledging the things that we do well as a team or field. We have advanced in many ways and aim to influence not only our organisation but also on national and international levels. We are present in training the new workforce (teaching on doctoral programmes in educational psychology and clinical psychology, and masters programmes in paediatric neuropsychology); we have developed organisation-wide mandatory psychosocial training (i.e., SPECS) and regularly present at conferences; and we also try to co-produce new developments with experts by experience and recruit our workforce with their help.

Conclusion

We are facing a time of change within the field of paediatric neurorehabilitation and acquired brain injury. The socio-political climate is such that attention is being given to greater integration, cross-departmental working, and the need to recognise the often hidden and invisible nature of ABI. This brings opportunities for action and greater attention to ASPs and their interaction with ABI. We have the potential to create meaningful change for CYPF living with ABI and to influence the systems that surround them.

This chapter has drawn our attention to those areas that are within our consciousness and to the inequities that are still unspoken or outside of our awareness. We have named both strengths and limitations in our service delivery and have acknowledged the bias within the foundations upon which our 'evidence-led' practice is based.

Through sharing their stories and experiences, CYPF have highlighted a conscious awareness of ASPs. They shared descriptions of the challenges they meet due to lack of awareness and understanding of ABI as well as the invisibility of their hidden needs. They also articulated the juxtaposition of having to mask their hidden needs and protect them as they connect to pre-injury identities, avoid stigma, and strive for equal opportunities in the workplace/school or acceptance from their peers. This reflects an awareness of the society they live in. CYPF are mindful of narratives of deficits and the challenges faced by those who need support. They were also seen to draw great strength from spiritual and cultural narratives of acceptance, love, and connection. The question therefore remains: What would non-ableist and non-Western approaches to rehabilitation look like? What do our CYPF need to achieve meaningful participation? Are the systems around them ready to change and respond to non-ableist approaches?

Mosleh (2019) highlights how rehabilitation has the potential to reinforce a notion of an 'ideal state or body' and, in turn, limits an ability to support people with disability due to perceptions of disability being within the individual. We acknowledge the need to look beyond the individual, challenge discourses that exist within society, and comprehend the impact of interacting systems and socio-political climates around the CYPF. We need to truly understand the lived experience of our CYP to promote meaningful participation and move away from ableist views of recovery of skills.

To do this we must enter into open communication with our CYPF in order to co-produce services and interventions in rehabilitation that truly reflect their goals and wishes. We should aim to facilitate participation and adaptation beyond the individual and to create opportunities within the system. We must also use our position and power to encourage national decision makers to explore alternative ways of designing services and creating models of delivery that are responsive and proactive in accordance with the lived experience of CYPF.

We need to be less 'localised' within our own fields and professional literature. For example, we saw that other fields exist that we were not aware of previously, such as 'Critical Rehabilitation', and we predict that many more will exist that could supply crucial ways of thinking to address our common dilemmas. We need to form our own foundational 'connectome' that links other fields, professions, and stakeholders.

Summary

Our Intentions for the Future

- ASPs remain a source of systemic disability that are within our gift to change. We will commit to talking about ASPs with CYPF, referrers, future service providers, and government bodies in order to challenge and openly address issues of intersectionality and promote equity across the system.
- We will commit to exploring privilege within research to understand how some groups may have advantages over others in an exponential pathway.
- Agents of advocacy and change are potentially present at all layers surrounding a CYPF. We will continue to mentalise CYPF's lived experience by listening and responding to what they tell us, taking the time to hear their wishes and feelings and to collaboratively promote authentically meaningful participation in rehabilitation.
- We will remain committed to reflexive practice, exploring our beliefs, judgements, and practices, which may be known or potentially unspoken, holding ourselves accountable and being accountable to our service users.
- We must commit ourselves to developing an evidence base that brings attention to the unsaid or unspoken narratives within the field as well as the questions that CYPF feel warrant attention to ensure our research is representative of the vast numbers of CYPF living with ABI.
- We need to acknowledge that CYP require advocates to ensure their voices are heard. The field is dominated by adult literature, which has the power to influence models and systems of service delivery. Children's voices also need to be heard. They can't be quietened or ignored, and it shouldn't remain the responsibility of their family/carers to bring the need for change to the attention of powerful social, political, and economic systems. We all need to do more to represent the developmental context that CYP face, hear their voices, and show them we are listening through positive action and change.

- Finally, we will make a commitment to exploring non-Western, non-ableist approaches to rehabilitation in order to understand how this might influence our models of service delivery and personal biases in therapeutic interventions.

References

All-Party Parliamentary Group on Acquired Brain Injury. (2018). *Acquired brain injury and neurorehabilitation: Time for change.* Available at: https://cdn.ymaws.com/ukabif.org.uk/resource/resmgr/campaigns/appg-abi_report_time-for-cha.pdf.

Anda, R. F., Butchart, A., Felitti, V. J., & Brown, D. W. (2010). Building a framework for global surveillance of the public health implications of adverse childhood experiences. *American Journal of Preventive Medicine, 39*(1), 93–98.

Anderson, V., Catroppa, C., Morse, S., Haritou, F., & Rosenfeld, J. (2005). Functional plasticity or vulnerability after early brain injury? *Pediatrics, 116*(6), 1374–1382.

Autism Act (2009). UK Public General Acts. *The National Archives.* Retrieved from: https://www.legislation.gov.uk/ukpga/2009/15/contents/enacted.

Bronfenbrenner, U. (1979). *The ecology of human development: Experiments by nature and design.* Cambridge, MA: Harvard University Press.

Dye, H. (2018). The impact and long-term effects of childhood trauma. *Journal of Human Behavior in the Social Environment, 28*(3), 381–392.

Forsyth, R., & Kirkham, F. (2012). Predicting outcome after childhood brain injury. *Canadian Medical Association Journal, 184*(11), 1257–1264.

Gormley, M., Devanaboyina, M., Andelic, N., Røe, C., Seel, R. T., & Lu, J. (2019). Long-term employment outcomes following moderate to severe traumatic brain injury: A systematic review and meta-analysis. *Brain Injury, 33*(13–14), 1567–1580.

Jim, J., & Norton, B. (2015). *'SPECS': A psychosocial training package for staff working in paediatric acquired brain injury.* 11th World congress on brain injury: Brain injury from cell to society, 2016. International Brain Injury Association (IBIA), The Hague, The Netherlands.

Katz-Leurer, M., Rotem, H., Keren, O., & Meyer, S. (2010). Recreational physical activities among children with a history of severe traumatic brain injury. *Brain Injury, 24*(13–14), 1561–1567.

Keetley, R., Westwater-Wood, S., & Manning, J. C. (2021). Exploring participation after paediatric acquired brain injury. *Journal of Child Health Care, 25*(1), 81–92.

Lyons, S., Whyte, K., Stephens, R., & Townsend, H. (2020). *Developmental Trauma Close Up.* Beacon House Therapeutic Services & Trauma Team. Available at: https://beaconhouse.org.uk/wp-content/uploads/2020/02/Developmental-Trauma-Close-Up-Revised-Jan-2020.pdf.

Miller, A. B., Esposito-Smythers, C., Weismoore, J. T., & Renshaw, K. D. (2013). The Relation Between Child Maltreatment and Adolescent Suicidal Behavior: A Systematic Review and Critical Examination of the Literature. *Clinical Child and Family Psychology Review, 16*(2), 146–172.

Mosleh, D. (2019). Critical Disability Studies With Rehabilitation: Re-thinking the human in rehabilitation research and practice. *Journal of Humanities in Rehabilitation*, Fall. Retrieved from: https://www.jhrehab.org/2019/11/14/ making-the-case-for-critical-disability-studies-with-rehabilitation-sciences.

NASEN and the Child Brain Injury Trust. (2018). *Childhood Acquired Brain Injury: The hidden disability*. nasen. Available at: https://childbraininjurytrust. org.uk/wp-content/uploads/2018/11/ABI-Mini-Guide.pdf.

NICE (National Institute for Health and Care Excellence). (2014). *Briefing Paper: Head Injury*. Available at: https://www.nice.org.uk/guidance/qs74/documents/ head-injury-briefing-paper2.

Odacı, H., & Çelik, Ç. B. (2020). The Role of Traumatic Childhood Experiences in Predicting a Disposition to Risk-Taking and Aggression in Turkish University Students. *Journal of Interpersonal Violence*, *35*(9–10), 1998–2011.

Raby, C., & Jones, F. (2016). Identifying risks for male street gang affiliation: A systematic review and narrative synthesis. *The Journal of Forensic Psychiatry & Psychology*, *27*(5), 601–644.

van der Kolk, B. A. (2005). Developmental Trauma Disorder: Toward a rational diagnosis for children with complex trauma histories. *Psychiatric Annals*, *35*(5), 401–408.

Williams, H. (2012). *Repairing Shattered Lives: brain injury and its implications for criminal justice*. Barrow Cadbury Trust. Available at: https://barrowcadbury. org.uk/wp-content/uploads/2012/11/Repairing-Shattered-Lives_Report.pdf.

Willmott, C., Ponsford, J., Downing, M., & Carty, M. (2014). Frequency and quality of return to study following traumatic brain injury. *The Journal of Head Trauma Rehabilitation*, *29*(3), 248–256.

Yeates, K. O., Taylor, H. G., Walz, N. C., Stancin, T., & Wade, S. L. (2010). The family environment as a moderator of psychosocial outcomes following traumatic brain injury in young children. *Neuropsychology*, *24*(3), 345–356.

Youth Justice Board and Ministry of Justice. (2021). *Youth Justice Statistics 2019/20 England and Wales: Statistics Bulletin*. Ministry of Justice. Available at: https://assets.publishing.service.gov.uk/government/uploads/system/ uploads/attachment_data/file/956621/youth-justice-statistics-2019-2020.pdf.

Part 3

Inclusion and the
Neuropsychological Setting

6 RACE-L Framework

Carrying Out Multicultural Neuropsychological Assessments

Sheeba Ehsan

Introduction

Britain is an ethnically diverse society; ethnic minorities make up 14% of the United Kingdom (UK) (Office for National Statistics, 2018). Under the Equality Act 2010, the UK government has a strong commitment to equality, and it is illegal to refuse certain rights on the grounds of race (Race Relations Act 1968, 2011). Therefore, services such as hospitals and immigration and social welfare systems must make sure they have the appropriate processes in place when working with ethnic minority populations (e.g., interpreters).

Within the profession and practice of psychology in the UK, protests following the racially motivated murder of George Floyd have pushed the British Psychological Society (BPS) to closely examine its relationship with institutional racism (Bajwa, 2020). The BPS has also been compelled to reflect on its roots and the system of White supremacy within UK clinical psychology training (Bajwa, 2020). The field of clinical neuropsychology has evolved due to developments in neurosciences (Roalf & Gur, 2017); however, consideration of culture and language within the profession are still in its infancy (Puente et al., 2013). This has led to privileging Whiteness, discriminating against non-Western forms of assessment, and perhaps misinforming diagnosis and treatment (Cory, 2020). In addition, there are White culturally and linguistically diverse populations within the UK for whom standard neuropsychology measures may not fit. It is important to consider assessment more broadly whilst incorporating factors such as culture and language to ensure that individuals from all ethnic groups have equal access to neuropsychology services.

Cognitive Risk Factors

Minority groups are at a higher risk of medical conditions associated with cognitive impairments, such as stroke and diabetes mellitus (Noble et al., 2012; Stronks et al., 2013; Trimble & Morgenstern, 2008). It is vital that cognitive assessments are accurate, as iatrogenic risk associated with misconceptions of being brain damaged is well documented amongst combat veterans with cognitive complaints (Roth & Spencer, 2013) as

DOI: 10.4324/9781003309819-9

well as in mild brain injury (Newcombe et al., 1994). The iatrogenic risk associated with surgical interventions for refractory epilepsy has also been well documented, and the role of neuropsychological assessment is established as important in calculating cognitive risk (Hermann et al., 2017). During the COVID-19 pandemic, minority ethnic groups were highlighted as at a higher risk of infection (Khunti et al, 2020) and there were adverse outcomes associated with long COVID (Naidu et al., 2021).

Multicultural Neuropsychological Test Application and Bias

The goal of any neuropsychological assessment is to be able to measure how well an individual's brain is functioning further to an organic process (e.g., dementia) or injury (e.g., traumatic brain injury); assessments aim to measure the extent of change from what is normal for that individual. This is achieved by using performance-based test batteries, which tap into specific domains (e.g., memory, language, IQ (Harvey, 2019)) and can then inform diagnosis, treatment, functional recovery, and rehabilitation. The assessment process has been heavily scrutinised, as it relies on psychometric tests which are developed and validated for use with Western or European populations (Ardila, 1998; Fernández & Evans, 2022). This presents a challenge for clinical neuropsychology services when assessing anybody from a non-dominant minority group.

The topic of IQ heritability and race differences in IQ has a controversial history (Colman, 2016). Poor performance on neuropsychological tests by ethnic minorities has been well documented (Rushton & Jensen, 2005) and may be due to a multitude of factors, including the normative data utilised (Werry et al., 2019) and the cultural content of the test instrument if it was designed and validated for use with a non-ethnic-minority group (Fernández & Abe, 2017).

It has also been proposed that brain function and development is highly culturally mediated, as our behaviour is highly dependent on what is normal to us as individuals, e.g., values, attitudes, etiquettes, etc. (Fernández & Abe, 2017). Van de Vijver and Tanzer (2004) presented the ideas of construct, method, and item biases, which have been applied in the context of neuropsychological testing to raise awareness of issues that require addressing (Fernández & Evans, 2022; Fernández & Abe, 2017). It is also important to recognise the possibility of a wider systemic and institutional bias. The possibility of clinician bias can be minimised by increasing self-awareness; this is important in the assessment process (Franzen et al., 2021). This may include cultural or racial identity, position of privilege, values, and how to be mindful of these through the assessment. It is the groundwork for training, education, and supervision and a valuable tool in addressing preconceived notions, racial bias, or cultural stereotypes (Ortiz & Lella, 2005).

When working with minority ethnic groups, several factors may pose a challenge for the clinician. Firstly, variables such as familiarity and proficiency in the assessment are often dependent on test validity. Proficiency is also dependent on training received around wider factors which influence assessments. Other factors include language, literacy, education, culture, and test sensitivity to these factors. The clinician has a choice as to whether to look for culturally fair tests developed in the individual's native culture and language, adapt tests, or develop them from scratch, and the following factors are crucial.

Factors Beyond Western Psychometrics

Race and Ethnicity

The importance of race-based normative data to improve the validity of neuropsychological tests has been highlighted (Gasquoine, 2009; Manly, 2005). Race and ethnicity are constructs related to human identity. Race is used to capture the values we ascribe to ourselves or others based on physical features, ancestry, and geographical origins (Bhopal, 1998). The construct of race can add value to interpretation of test scores by facilitating a deeper understanding of more meaningful variables, e.g., quality of education.

Ethnicity relates to an individual's ancestral roots embedded in cultural traditions, religion, race, and language (Bhopal, 1998). Race and ethnicity overlap and are used synonymously (Bhopal, 1998). They are known as controversial variables as 'biological/innate based definitions' have attributed group differences between IQ and race to genetic factors (Markus, 2008). Such spurious information is often the root cause for systems denying equality and disadvantaging people (Markus, 2008). To be ethno-culturally responsive, we need to be 'open to the other'; therefore, it is helpful to understand cultural competency as a process rather than the finished product. Cultural humility, as discussed in Chapter 11, encourages the neuropsychologist to maintain an interpersonal stance that is other-oriented (or open to the other) in relation to aspects of cultural identity that are most important to the person (Hook at cl., 2013). If the neuropsychologist applies an interpersonal stance which is genuinely curious, this can potentially lead them to take important variables into account and foster a stronger alliance in the assessment situation.

Language

Healthcare providers are under pressure to meet the needs of the UK's increasingly diverse population. In the UK between one in five and one in ten people do not speak English as their first language (Office of National Statistics, 2011a, 2011b). One of the challenges for clinical neuropsychology becoming ethno-culturally responsive is the lack of availability of cross-linguistic assessments and normative data in those languages (Manly, 2008). Language usage varies greatly according to the culture and subculture, which can greatly impact dialect and is moderated by educational ability (Pérez-Arce, 1999).

Language function is distributed across neuronal networks in the brain and can be observed using Functional Magnetic Resonance Imaging (fMRI) (Luckett et al., 2020). It has been reported that during language processing, different languages are associated with various brain activations (Paulesu et al., 2000). FMRI studies of bilinguals across closely similar spoken languages (yet distinct in writing), e.g., Hindi and Urdu, suggest that crucial areas (middle and superior frontal regions) for processing of orthography and graphemic complexity are found for one (Urdu) but not the other (Hindi) (Kumar, 2014). Neurocognitive models of brain function in bilinguals suggest that functional organisation is mediated by factors such as age of acquisition (Hull & Vaid, 2007). Languages vary greatly in terms of phonology, lexicon, grammar, pragmatic, and reading systems (Ardila, 2007). It is suggested that bilingualism elicits several neuroanatomical changes (Taylor et al., 2022); clinically, this suggests caution to any assumptions which may be drawn based on prior neuroanatomical knowledge. The literature highlights the importance of understanding language diversity across cultures to inform cultural assessments.

Culture

Culture has been defined as the collection of values, attitudes, traditions, behaviours, and language specific to a group of individuals, which are transmitted across generations (Matsumoto, 1994). Culture is understood to be a socially constructed and fluid concept (Jugert et al., 2021; Bhopal, 2004). Culture is thought to provide us with explicit models of thinking and relating to the world, which is represented on test performance (Ardila, 1995) and can be a moderating factor in neuropsychological test performance (Ardila, 1993, 1995; Nell, 1999). Cultural differences in performance on perceptual judgment and memory tasks (Ji et al., 2000; Nisbett & Masuda, 2003) and visual information processing have been reported (Goto et al., 2010). Cultural bias is any factor during the assessment process which results in systemic differences in performance between the individual's culture and the majority culture, e.g., assessment setting, test material/norms, appropriateness of test stimuli/items/terms (Ortiz & Leila, 2005), and psychological constructs (Ardila, 2005).

Within the testing situation, we are interested in any factors which would impact performance due to the variable culture, e.g., values such as deference to authority, the importance of 'keeping face', modesty, communication style, eye contact, etc. Within the assessment context, culture may affect aspects of response style, speed, or even motivation (Ortiz & Lella, 2005). For example, to avoid loss of face, Asian Americans might evade guessing an answer or expanding on responses or giving self-assured statements (Zane & Yeh, 2002). A modest individual may say 'I don't know' in response to a question out of modesty or a lack of confidence, rather than not knowing (Zane & Yeh, 2002).

Acculturation

Acculturation defines the process which occurs when an individual or groups of people transition from living a lifestyle of their own culture to moving into one that is different to their own (Arends-Tóth & Van de Vijver, 2006). Acculturation is thought to correlate with performance on neuropsychological measures (Baird et al., 2007).

To achieve assessments in which the impact of culture is minimised, we need to cultivate ethno-sensitivity within our materials, processes, and clinicians, as discussed below.

Culturally Guided Assessments

The presentation of ethnic minorities has unsurprisingly presented a challenge during the cognitive assessment process. Individuals from ethnic minority backgrounds are at risk of neurological conditions and present to services across the UK, albeit at a lesser pace than their White counterparts (Dunning & Teager, 2020). If barriers to accessing services (Mirza et al., 2021) are addressed, then we are likely to have increased numbers of individuals who we are not fit to assess. Providing an equitable and culturally guided neuropsychology service is challenging. The challenges are also in avoiding practices based on assumptions, e.g., the assumption that non-verbal tests are culturally fair (Gonthier, 2022). There is a call for the urgent need to adapt existing tests or develop new tests (Franzen et al., 2021).

Meeting individuals' needs and continuing to provide a neuropsychological service are two different ideologies; to meet the needs of a diverse population, we need a change in the core practices and tools of the trade. To continue to provide a service, we can lift the standard by being more aware of all the factors beyond Western psychometrics. Daryl Fujii (2016) provides in-depth guidelines on how to achieve a robust cross-cultural assessment in his book. Here the author presents guidelines from the experience of interpreter-mediated assessments in conjunction with a formulation diagram developed to facilitate the assessment process.

Cross-Cultural Testing: Clinical Reflections and Practical Solutions

Cross-cultural tests are tests which have been developed with culture in mind, therefore they can be applied within different cultural settings. There are a limited number of tests available, which certainly does not meet the demands of the UK with its ever-changing population becoming more and more diverse. The tables below (Tables 6.1 and 6.2) show how language differences can be addressed to improve the validity of neuropsychological assessments.

The interpretation of test material provides a challenge, especially when one considers types of biases:

- Method bias: Does changing the language in which a test is administered change what it is measuring?
- Construct bias: Is the cognitive construct being measured universally expressed in the same way?

Table 6.1 Interpreter-Facilitated Assessment

Processes and possible difficulties in the assessment process	Facilitators of assessment
Language match	• It is vital that the interpreter is matched to client, languages may have many dialects or local variations. The closer the match the better the engagement (a shared sense of knowing); this is also beneficial as the interpreter may be able to part cultural knowledge pertinent to the assessment.
Guidance	• There is key guidance from the BPS which can help shape assessments through interpreters. Some of the key points to note for neuropsychology assessments start by highlighting the difference between standard interpretation and that required for an effective neuropsychology assessment. Think about this e.g., plan with a pre session.
Socialisation	• Training should be provided to socialise the interpreter to the goal of the assessment and the need for stricter adherence during a testing situation. For example, the interpreter should not provide any clarification on an instruction without discussion with the examiner. The emphasis being that the neuropsychological examination can guide diagnostics which has implications. Model with real-life situations.
Interpreter bias	• All communication is important and required, i.e. not a summary of what was discussed. Encourage audio recording of responses and score the results together.
Boundaries	• Clarification of role and stance is paramount. Boundaries are important but allow the interpreter to be curious in the pre-session.
Process bias	• The same interpreter should be used for all sessions.
Process bias	• Consider how broader factors such as history of stigmatisation and oppression may influence the three people during the assessment process. Allow for a debrief and test scoring session.

Table 6.2 Interpreter-Assisted Test Adaptation

Processes and possible difficulties in the assessment process	Facilitators of assessment
Cultural bias	• Meet with the interpreter in advance of the assessment session and talk some of these factors through. Use your assessment to guide the discussion.
Cultural bias	• Allow extra time to understand if there is shared terminology between the two languages.
Construct bias	• Think about the individual items on more language heavy assessments (e.g., naming tests, comprehension, similarities, verbal memory tests, etc.). Can these be adjusted?
Translation	• Once the material has been discussed the process of translation can take place; this can often lead to items being adapted to match the patient's culture e.g., changing an item or word for an equivalent. Where possible the clinician should gain as much knowledge about the individual's culture to help guide the item selection. The item should be matched for difficulty level.
Preparation	• Translation of test instructions and test items should be done in advance of the session. Forms with the translated material (phonetically) should be available for the assessor to follow and guide the assessment.
Scoring and Reporting	• When scoring allow for adjustments based on cultural considerations. Report your results transparently with reference to adaptations and limitations.

• Instrument bias: Is the patient familiar with the idea of assessment? (In non-educated populations, this may be the individual's first encounter with assessment.)

Neuropsychologists are trained to think about factors such as age, gender, and educational influences on performance. From the literature reviewed, factors such as ethnicity and culture are also important. Figures 6.1 and 6.2 are designed to provide a framework for this process.

A key aspect is to consider the training needs of any individuals delivering neuropsychological assessment. There are no current competency guidelines for neuropsychologists conducting cross-cultural assessments in the UK. However, broader guidelines for working with diversity are available (American Psychological Association, 2010). Key factors to consider during the assessment and case conceptualisation include Race, Acculturation, Culture, Ethnicity, and Language, or RACE-L (see Figures 6.1 and 6.2).

RACE-L principles are guided by a stance of cultural humility and influenced by the individual's environmental experience. The assessor

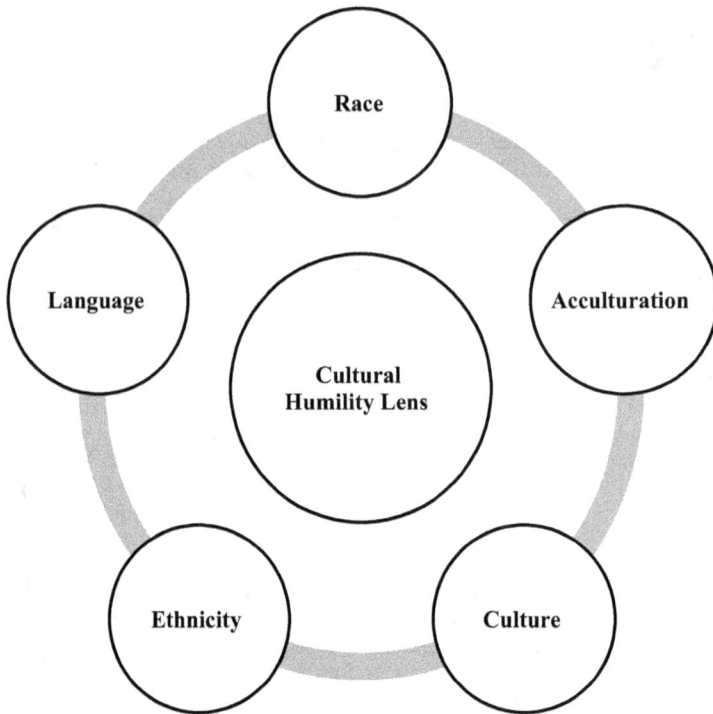

Figure 6.1 RACE-L Model for Guiding Cross-Cultural Assessment and Formulation

is encouraged to think about the formulation points fluidly, e.g., What caused the person to leave their country? or How might the individual's experience(s) interplay with the assessment? The RACE-L themes guide the assessment by considering individual and cultural diversity and context.

What Can Be Achieved within our Current Practices?

Below are case examples of how the RACE-L model can be applied to guide case conceptualisation. All results were interpreted with caution, and a thorough assessment meant any threats to validity of test scores were apparent. The clinician relied on theoretical knowledge of neuropsychology for interpretation of all test material.

Case Study 1

A 20-year-old male presented to a regional neuropsychology service further to a traumatic brain injury (TBI). He was involved in a road traffic accident as a cyclist, which resulted in a traumatic subdural and

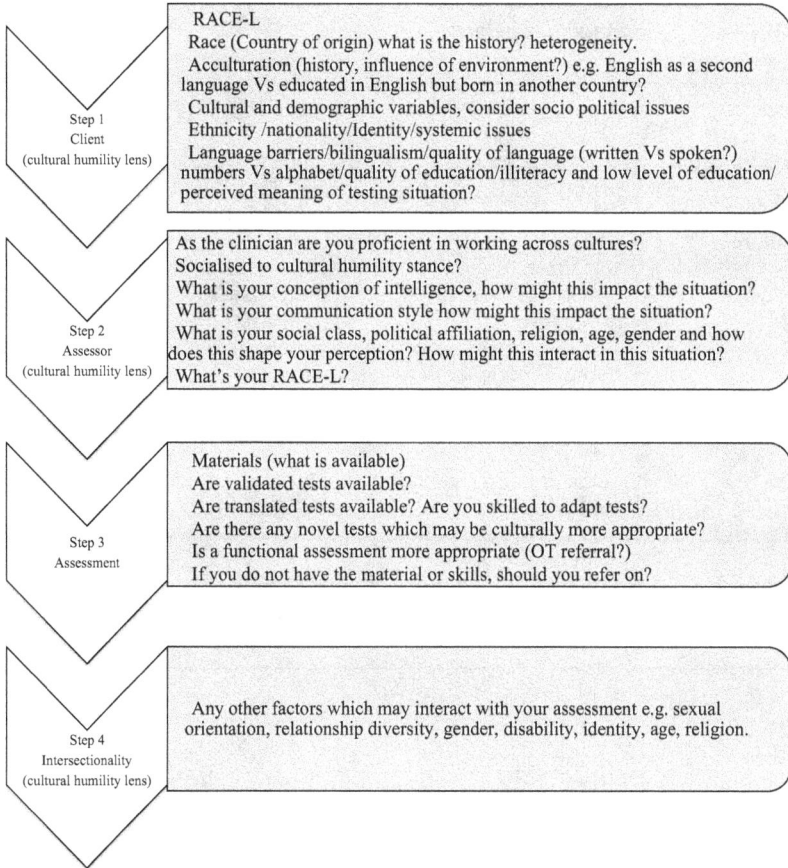

Step 1
Client
(cultural humility lens)

RACE-L
Race (Country of origin) what is the history? heterogeneity.
Acculturation (history, influence of environment?) e.g. English as a second language Vs educated in English but born in another country?
Cultural and demographic variables, consider socio political issues
Ethnicity /nationality/Identity/systemic issues
Language barriers/bilingualism/quality of language (written Vs spoken?) numbers Vs alphabet/quality of education/illiteracy and low level of education/ perceived meaning of testing situation?

Step 2
Assessor
(cultural humility lens)

As the clinician are you proficient in working across cultures?
Socialised to cultural humility stance?
What is your conception of intelligence, how might this impact the situation?
What is your communication style how might this impact the situation?
What is your social class, political affiliation, religion, age, gender and how does this shape your perception? How might this interact in this situation?
What's your RACE-L?

Step 3
Assessment

Materials (what is available)
Are validated tests available?
Are translated tests available? Are you skilled to adapt tests?
Are there any novel tests which may be culturally more appropriate?
Is a functional assessment more appropriate (OT referral?)
If you do not have the material or skills, should you refer on?

Step 4
Intersectionality
(cultural humility lens)

Any other factors which may interact with your assessment e.g. sexual orientation, relationship diversity, gender, disability, identity, age, religion.

Figure 6.2 RACE-L Model for Guiding Cross-Cultural Assessment and Formulation

subarachnoid haemorrhage and mandibular fracture. He was treated for his injuries with an inpatient stay and was discharged with no community follow-up. He presented to neuropsychology services with memory and mood difficulties. He was assessed by the clinical neuropsychologist in his first language (Punjabi); however, on the referral it did indicate he spoke Hindi (a common mistake and assumption).

This gentleman was identified as having little or no social support. He said that he was financially dependent on his family, and whilst in hospital he had been the target of financial abuse by a 'friend' in the UK. He was not entitled to any funds or extra support from the government. There was a change of role and identity for him.

Table 6.3 Case Study 1

RACE-L Model	Formulation points	
Race	Asian, born in Pakistan.	Ancestors all from Pakistan and farmers.
Acculturation	6 months in the UK prior to TBI.	First male to leave his village and come to the UK to study and support his family.
Culture	Native Pakistani, socialised to the UK only for 6months, expectation to support family back home, experience of prejudice, emotional expression seen as a weakness. Passive to authority, less likely to challenge.	No schooling in his village; parents/ ancestors have their own land and the male's role is hands on agriculture. Not socialised to any testing situation. Strong faith system Not socialised to recognising emotions, emotional issues more likely to manifest as physical symptoms.
Ethnicity	Minority group with no local family support.	
Language	No English language, first language Punjabi.	Punjabi speaking from a village in Pakistan, local dialect different from the city.

Plan

The plan was to involve his friends and family to gain further information and corroborate the information provided. The main pressing issue was identified as low mood.

Clinical Context

Intrapersonal: It was important to recognise the power imbalance and my identity as an Asian female in a position of authority. Interpersonal: It was important to acknowledge that he had no experience of any formal testing or schooling.

Assessment and Intervention

A search was carried out for assessments in his native language. There were limited resources. The clinician then adapted test material, informed by the case conceptualisation. The Hospital Anxiety Depression Scale (HADS) was translated. Issues with low mood were highlighted. Physical symptoms were also elicited, for example, fatigue, broken sleep, pains in his face and body, and dizzy spells on climbing stairs. His self-report indicated poor memory and reduced motivation. Further assessment highlighted psychological post-trauma symptoms and lack of support. The clinical work focused on psychoeducation; he was socialised to adapted cognitive behavioural intervention and strategies for managing distress alongside antidepressants prescribed by his GP. His self-reported memory difficulties stabilised as psychological difficulties improved; therefore, no cognitive assessment was required.

Reflection

The importance of a thorough assessment in the patient's native language was highlighted. This shaped and informed the clinician's plan for further assessment and treatment. If a cognitive assessment was conducted, it would have been difficult to interpret due to the multitude of difficulties. Therefore, it was important to engage in mindful/active listening and to ask open-ended questions to assess priority. By doing this, the clinician was able to see if it made a difference to other areas of function. An understanding of intersectionality, psychological processes involved in living with disability, and the change of identity were helpful tools to help navigate the distress.

In this example, the individual, with no clear person to advocate, was lost to community follow-up. There may be many people in this position due to gaps in service provision and lack of follow-up. The patient's neurorehabilitation and emotional needs remained unmet at discharge, perhaps due to a focus on physical recovery and a lack of understanding of his emotional needs.

Case Study 2

A 22-year-old female was referred to a regional neuropsychology service for an assessment further to her diagnosis of epilepsy. Her seizures began in adulthood. A scan of her brain had identified a region which was likely contributing to her seizures; therefore, she was being considered for surgery. She was bilingual; however, she was tested in English, as she had been educated in English. This decision was made further to a thorough assessment.

This female was identified as having limited family support, which would be an important factor to consider if this person was to undergo surgery. She had been ostracised by her community in Africa, as she was labelled as possessed by an evil spirit due to her seizures. She had been exposed to alternative doctors and trialled ritualistic treatments. This experience had led her to experience feelings of shame and made her less likely to share her distress with her current community.

Plan

Cognitive assessment and mood screen in English.

Table 6.4 Case Study 4

RACE-L Model	Formulation points	
Race	African Somali, born in North Africa.	
Acculturation	Came to the UK as an adult prior to epilepsy diagnosis. Recalls lapses in her attention from her teens.	Educated in the UK system. Worked in UK. Fear of being ostracised by local community, may be less likely to share distress. Poor support system.
Culture	Native African, socialised to the UK 5 years, sought alternative practices in the past. Experience of prejudice related to identity and illness. Belief system externalising illness, e.g. spirit possession. Passive to authority, less likely to challenge.	Educated through the education system in Africa, socialised to learning and test situations. Strong faith system, limited family support due to illness perception of dominant culture.
Ethnicity	Minority, with experience of being ostracised by own community group (stigma).	
Language	Can be tested in English.	Fluent in Swahili in addition to English. Many languages spoken in Africa.

Clinical Context

Intrapersonal: It was important to recognise the power imbalance and my identity as an Asian female in a position of authority and to understand cultural influences on perception and practices.

Assessment and Intervention

All psychometric tests were delivered in English. An interesting point to note is that she was educated to degree level, but her predicted premorbid ability was in the low average range. This was not consistent with her educational background. Further, the results of her memory assessment suggested that the side of her brain which was being considered for surgery was stronger (i.e., stronger verbal memory versus nonverbal memory). Her performance on the language tests (which would include culturally biased items) was also poor. This highlighted the impact of culture and the limitations of the tests utilised even when the person does speak English as a second language.

Intervention work mainly focused on psychoeducation. The assessment also highlighted low mood, low confidence, and a lack of support and understanding. Compassion-focussed therapy sessions were helpful to work with issues of shame and self-criticism.

Case Study 3

A 43-year-old male was referred to a regional neuropsychology service for a neuropsychological assessment further to his diagnosis of a brain tumour following a recent seizure. He was an inpatient at the time of referral. A brain scan had demonstrated a lesion on the left posterior temporal region, an area fundamental for language skills, such as word retrieval (Hope & Price, 2016). Therefore, a procedure known as awake craniotomy was recommended; the patient is kept awake during surgery and undergoes a continuous clinical assessment (Hall et al., 2021). The surgeon uses intraoperative direct electrical stimulation (DES) to map eloquent brain areas, thus allowing maximum safe removal of the tumour (Szelényi et al., 2010). During the clinical assessment it was established that the patient spoke some English, but his primary language was Cantonese. The decision was made to conduct the assessment and the awake craniotomy in Cantonese. The neuropsychologist searched the literature and liaised with senior clinicians throughout the UK to establish whether any tests were available in the person's native language. The neuropsychologist gained a good understanding of the patient's language abilities, e.g., speaking, comprehension, writing, numeracy, and literacy abilities. The neuropsychologist was able to speak to his wife and gain a good understanding of any baseline cognitive issues.

Plan

The cognitive assessment was conducted in Cantonese and English using adapted versions of standardised tests and the interpreter service. In discussion with the neurosurgeon, an intraoperative battery of naming, counting, and repetitio was decided on. The plan was to establish a cognitive baseline prior to surgery in an inpatient setting.

Clinical Context

Intrapersonal: It was important to recognise the power imbalance and my identity as an Asian female in a position of authority and gain a shared understanding of the diagnosis and treatment plan. The relationship is paramount for an awake craniotomy. This gentleman was referred as an inpatient, and the time to surgery was imminent; therefore, a shorter assessment was more realistic. The individual's language function would require monitoring during the awake surgery; therefore,

Table 6.5 Case Study 3

RACE-L Model	Formulation points
Race	*Asian, born in Hong Kong.*
Acculturation	Came to the UK aged 17, lived with his family including one brother who was in the UK. He went to college for 2 years on a student Visa, then he met his wife and got married (British Chinese wife). Own business in the UK (seen as achievement), new identity. He was able to use English language in the takeaway business, e.g. to take customer orders, but he mentioned that this raised his anxiety.
Culture	Native Chinese. He attended school in his home country. He was more likely to express emotions as somatic. His wife did all household tasks at home (important to record in his notes for any occupational therapy assessments). He had been to see a Chinese doctor (herbalist). There was a sense of responsibility for his family back home and in the UK.
Ethnicity	Minority group belonging to Han Chinese. Different norms, values and beliefs around health, and health care. May impact sense of safety in a Western medicine/health care system.
Language	Main language Cantonese spoken at home. He went to college in the UK and completed basic level English qualification. Prefers to use first language where possible. Some knowledge of testing practices in the UK e.g., studied to ESOL level. Can count in both English and Cantonese. Familiar with the English alphabet. Prefers Cantonese.

the role of the interpreter was paramount in facilitating this. It was important that the neuropsychologist built a shared understanding with the interpreter.

Assessment and Intervention

Self-reported periods of frustration and concentration lapses were highlighted. The assessment focussed on socialising the patient to the reasons for assessing at baseline and making sure this was understood and consented to. All tests, where possible, were adapted and delivered in Cantonese. The interpreter service was used alongside the clinician's knowledge of the language (time spent listening to the phonetic sounds in Cantonese and writing these down in English for all language-based tests). Some tests were delivered in English only, e.g., digit span, whilst some tests were delivered in both English and Cantonese, e.g., semantic fluency section. The results of his assessment highlighted no difficulties (Repeatable Battery for the Assessment of Neuropsychological Status, RBANS); however, it was noted that he took longer to respond on the digit span (delivered in English). Interestingly, both the English and Cantonese semantic fluency scores were similar.

This patient was prepared for surgery utilising the same interpreter, and the neuropsychologist's confidence in the interpreter's accuracy was established.

Conclusion

In summary, this chapter provided the reader with an overview of challenges faced by neuropsychology services due to the rise of a multicultural society. The primary issues relevant to the clinical practice of cross-cultural testing were discussed. The current model of neuropsychological assessment in the UK was developed on a culture of high productivity, competitiveness, literacy, and speed, which represents the dominant Western culture. Western tests of intelligence and cognitive ability are biased in several ways, and the clinician is therefore placed in a possible discriminatory position. There is no real comparison between minority groups' performance on tests and the performance of those on whom the tests were normed. Furthermore, if a cognitive assessment is necessitated, everything must be done clinically to lessen the likelihood of bias, including:

- Conducting a thorough assessment guided by the RACE-L model (Figures 6.1 and 6.2) to ascertain the impact of culture and other important factors;
- Searching for appropriate tests which are normed for the individual being assessed;

- Taking the necessary steps to identify and train the appropriate interpreter, i.e., socialising to clinical neuropsychology; and
- Ensuring ethno-culturally informed assessment by embodying a position of cultural humility.

It would be beneficial for those developing tests to be mindful and aware of concepts which are outside of or beyond mainstream UK values. A collaborative approach which avoids race-based norms and instead supports a culturally sensitive assessment in diverse populations is favoured. In addition, neuropsychology trainees should be taught the importance of cultural and educational issues in relation to brain function.

References

American Psychological Association. (2010). *Ethical principles of psychologists and code of conduct.*

Ardila, A. (Ed.). (1993). On the origins of cognitive activity [Special issue]. *Behavioural Neurology, 6,* 71–74.

Ardila, A. (1995). Directions of research in cross-cultural neuropsychology. *Journal of Clinical and Experimental Neuropsychology, 17,* 143–150.

Ardila, A. (1998). A note of caution: Normative neuropsychological test performance: Effects of age, education, gender and ethnicity: A comment on Saykin et al. (1995). *Applied Neuropsychology, 5,* 51–53.

Ardila, A. (2005). Cultural values underlying psychometric cognitive testing. *Neuropsychology Review, 15,* 185–196.

Ardila, A. (2007). The impact of culture on neuropsychological test performance. In B. Uzzell, M. Pontón, & A. Ardila (Eds.), *International handbook of crosscultural neuropsychology* (pp. 23–45). Lawrence Erlbaum Associates.

Arends-Tóth, J. V., & Van de Vijver, F. J. R. (2006). Assessment of psychological acculturation. In D. L. Sam & J. W. Berry (Eds.), *The Cambridge handbook of acculturation psychology* (pp. 142–160). Cambridge University Press.

Baird, A., Ford., M., & Podell., K. (2007). Ethnic differences in functional and neuropsychological test performance in older adults. *Archives of Clinical Neuropsychology, 22,* 309–318.

Bajwa, S. (2020). Is the British Psychological Society institutionally racist? *BPS conference 2020.* https://www.bps.org.uk/blogs/chief-executive/british-psychological-society-institutionally-racist.

Bhopal, R. (1998). Spectre of racism in health and health care: Lessons from history and the United States. *BMJ (Clinical research ed.), 316*(7149), 1970–1973.

Bhopal, R. (2004). Glossary of terms relating to ethnicity and race: For reflection and debate. *Journal of Epidemiology & Community Health, 58*(6), 441–445.

Colman, A. M. (2016). Race differences in IQ: Hans Eysenck's contribution to the debate in the light of subsequent research. *Personality and Individual Differences, 103,* 182–189.

Cory, J. M. (2020). White privilege in neuropsychology: An "invisible knapsack" in need of unpacking? *The Clinical Neuropsychologist, 35*(2), 206–218.

Dunning, G., & Teager, A. (2020). An evaluation of ethnicity in a neuropsychology outpatient department. Paper presented at the Division of Clinical

Psychology (DCP) Annual Conference – 'Doing What Matters: Value-Driven Clinical Psychology in Action'.

Fernández, A. L., & Abe, J. (2017). Bias in cross-cultural neuropsychological testing: Problems and possible solutions. *Culture and Brain, 6*(1), 1–35.

Fernández, A. L., & Evans, J. (2022). *Understanding Cross-Cultural Neuropsychology: Science, Testing and Challenges.* Routledge.

Franzen, S., Papma, J. M., van den Berg, E., & Nielsen, T. R. (2021). Cross-cultural neuropsychological assessment in the European Union: A Delphi expert study. *Archives of Clinical Neuropsychology, 36*(5), 815–830. DOI: 10.1093/arclin/acaa083.

Fujii, D. (2016). *Conducting a culturally informed neuropsychological evaluation.* American Psychological Association. DOI: 10.1037/15958-000.

Gasquoine, P. G. (2009). Race-Norming of Neuropsychological Tests. *Neuropsychology Review, 19*(2), 250–262.

Gonthier, C. (2022). Cross-cultural differences in visuo-spatial processing and the culture-fairness of visuo-spatial intelligence tests: An integrative review and a model for matrices tasks. *Cognitive Research: Principles and Implications, 7*(1), 1–27.

Goto, S. G., Ando, Y., Huang, C., Yee, A., & Lewis, R. S. (2010). Cultural differences in the visual processing of meaning: Detecting incongruities between background and foreground objects using the N400. *Social Cognitive and Affective Neuroscience, 5*(2–3), 242–253.

Hall, S., Kabwama, S., Sadek, A.-R., Dando, A., Roach, J., Weidmann, C., & Grundy, P. (2021). Awake craniotomy for tumour resection: The safety and feasibility of a simple technique. *Interdisciplinary Neurosurgery, 24*, 101070. DOI: 10.1016/j.inat.2020.101070.

Harvey, P. D. (2019). Domains of cognition and their assessment. *Dialogues in Clinical Neuroscience, 21*(3), 227–237.

Hermann, B., Loring, D. W., & Wilson, S. (2017). Paradigm Shifts in the Neuropsychology of Epilepsy. *Journal of the International Neuropsychological Society, 23*(9–10), 791–805.

Hook, J. N., Davis, D. E., Owen, J., Worthington, E. L., & Utsey, S. O. (2013). Cultural humility: Measuring openness to culturally diverse clients. *Journal of Counselling Psychology, 60*(3), 353–366.

Hope, T. M. H., & Price, C. J. (2016). Why the left posterior inferior temporal lobe is needed for word finding. *Brain, 139*(11), 2823–2826.

Hull, R., & Vaid, J. (2007). Bilingual language lateralization: A meta-analytic tale of two hemispheres. *Neuropsychologia, 45*(9), 1987–2008.

Ji, L. J., Peng, K., & Nisbett, R. E. (2000). Culture, control, and perception of relationships in the environment. *Journal of Personality and Social Psychology, 78*(5), 943–955.

Jugert, P., Kaiser, M. J., Ialuna, F., & Civitillo, S. (2021). Researching race-ethnicity in race-mute Europe. *Infant and Child Development, 31*(1), e2260. DOI: 10.1002/icd.2260.

Khunti, K., Singh, A. K., Pareek, M., & Hanif, W. (2020). Is ethnicity linked to incidence or outcomes of covid-19? *BMJ, 369*(8243). DOI: 10.1136/bmj.m1548.

Kumar, U. (2014). Effect of orthography over neural regions in bilinguals: A view from neuroimaging. *Neuroscience Letters, 580*, 94–99.

Luckett, P., Lee, J. J., Park, K. Y., Dierker, D., Daniel, A. G. S., Seitzman, B. A., Hacker, C. D., Ances, B. M., Leuthardt, E. C., Snyder, A. Z., & Shimony, J.

S. (2020). Mapping of the language network with deep learning. *Frontiers in Neurology, 11,* 819. DOI: 10.3389/fneur.2020.00819.

Manly, J. J. (2005). Advantages and disadvantages of separate norms for African Americans. *The Clinical Neuropsychologist, 19*(2), 270–275.

Manly, J. J. (2008). Critical issues in cultural neuropsychology: Profit from diversity. *Neuropsychology Review, 18*(3), 179–183.

Markus, H. R. (2008). Pride, prejudice, and ambivalence: Toward a unified theory of race and ethnicity. *American Psychologist, 63*(8), 651–670.

Matsumoto, D. (1994). *Cultural influences on research methods and statistics.* Brooks/Cole.

Mirza, N., Vikram, A., Osmani, F., Kumar, N., Orakzai, S., Sharma, S., & Ehsan, S. (2021). Barriers and facilitators British ethnic minorities face when accessing neuropsychological services: A systematic review and qualitative analysis. Poster presented at the British Psychological Society annual conference: Positive adaptations: Psychological strengths.

Naidu, S. B., Shah, A. J., Saigal, A., Brill, S. E., Jarvis, H., Goldring, J. G., Wey, E., Miller, D., Abubakar, I., Hurst, J. R., Lipman, M., & Mandal, S. (2021). The impact of ethnicity on the long-term sequelae of COVID-19: Follow-up from the first and second waves in North London. *Thorax, 76*(Suppl 2), A141.

Nell, V. (1999). *Cross-Cultural Neuropsychological Assessment.* Psychology Press.

Newcombe, R., Rabbitt, P., & Briggs. M. (1994). Minor head injury: Pathophysiological or iatrogenic sequelae? *Journal of Neurology, Neurosurgery, and Psychiatry, 57,* 709–771.

Nisbett, R. E., & Masuda, T. (2003). Culture and point of view. *Proceedings of the National Academy of Sciences, 100*(19), 11163–11170.

Noble, J. M., Manly, J. J., Schupf, N., Tang, M.-X., & Luchsinger, J. A. (2012). Type 2 diabetes and ethnic disparities in cognitive impairment. *Ethnicity & Disease, 22*(1), 38–44.

Office for National Statistics. (2011a). 2011 Census: Key statistics for England and Wales, March 2011. *ons.gov.uk.* https://www.ons.gov.uk/census/2011census.

Office for National Statistics. (2011b). Language in England and Wales. *ons.gov. uk.* https://www.ons.gov.uk/peoplepopulationandcommunity/culturalidentity/language/articles/languageinenglandandwales/2013-03-04.

Office for National Statistics. (2018, August 1). Population of England and Wales. *GOV.UK.* https://www.ethnicity-facts-figures.service.gov.uk/uk-population-by-ethnicity/national-and-regional-populations/population-of-england-and-wales/latest.

Ortiz, S. O., & Lella, S. A. (2005). *Cross-Cultural Assessment.* SAGE Publications, Inc.

Paulesu, E., McCrory, E., Fazio, F., Menoncello, L., Brunswick, N., Cappa, S. F., Cotelli, M., Cossu, G., Corte, F., Lorusso, M., Pesenti, S., Gallagher, A., Perani, D., Price, C., Frith, C. D., & Frith, U. (2000). A cultural effect on brain function. *Nature Neuroscience, 3*(1), 91–96.

Pérez-Arce, P. (1999). The Influence of Culture on Cognition. *Archives of Clinical Neuropsychology, 14*(7), 581–592.

Puente, A. E., Perez-Garcia, M., Lopez, R. V., Hidalgo-Ruzzante, N. A., & Fasfous, A. F. (2013). Neuropsychological assessment of culturally and educationally dissimilar individuals. In F. A. Paniagua & A.-M. Yamada (Eds.),

Handbook of multicultural mental health: Assessment and treatment of diverse populations (pp. 225–241). Elsevier Academic Press.

Race Relations Act 1968. (2011). *Legislation.gov.uk.* https://www.legislation.gov.uk/ukpga/1968/71/enacted.

Roalf, D. R., & Gur, R. C. (2017). Functional brain imaging in neuropsychology over the past 25 years. *Neuropsychology, 31*(8), 954–971.

Roth, Y., & Spencer, R.J. (2013). Iatrogenic Risk in the Management of Mild Traumatic Brain Injury among Combat Veterans: A Case Illustration and Commentary. *International Journal of Physical Medicine and Rehabilitation, 1*, 1–7.

Rushton, J. P., & Jensen, A. R. (2005). Thirty years of research on race differences in cognitive ability. *Psychology, Public Policy, and Law, 11*(2), 235–294.

Stronks, K., Snijder, M. B., Peters, R. J., Prins, M., Schene, A. H., & Zwinderman, A. H. (2013). Unravelling the impact of ethnicity on health in Europe: The HELIUS study. *BMC Public Health, 13*(1), 402. DOI: 10.1186/1471-2458-13-402.

Szelényi, A., Bello, L., Duffau, H., Fava, E., Feigl, G. C., Galanda, M., Neuloh, G., Signorelli, F., & Sala, F. (2010). Intraoperative electrical stimulation in awake craniotomy: methodological aspects of current practice. *Neurosurgical Focus, 28*(2), E7.

Taylor, C., Hall, S., Manivannan, S., Mundil, N., & Border, S. (2022) The neuroanatomical consequences and pathological implications of bilingualism. *Journal of Anatomy, 240*, 410–427.

Trimble, B., & Morgenstern, L. B. (2008). Stroke in Minorities. *Neurologic Clinics, 26*(4), 1177–1190.

Van de Vijver, F., & Tanzer, N. K. (2004). Bias and equivalence in cross-cultural assessment: An overview. *European Review of Applied Psychology, 54*(2), 119–135.

Werry, A. E., Daniel, M., & Bergström, B. (2019). Group differences in normal neuropsychological test performance for older non-Hispanic White and Black/African American adults. *Neuropsychology, 33*(8), 1089–1100. DOI: 10.1037/neu0000579.

Zane, N., & Yeh, M. (2002). The use of culturally-based variables in assessment: Studies on loss of face. In K. S. Kurasaki, S. Okazaki, & S. Sue (Eds.), *Asian American mental health assessment theories and methods* (pp. 123–137). Kluwer Academic/Plenum.

7 Beyond the Index Injury

Creating Space for Race and Ethnicity in Personal Injury Neurorehabilitation Work

Shabnam Berry-Khan

Introduction

Across the globe in the 21st Century, research from any field of study largely supports the notion that White-majority populations fare better or have better outcomes than those with black or brown skin, termed here people of colour (POC). In the United Kingdom, it is becoming more accepted that conscious and unconscious race-related biases exist on many levels (West et al., 2021), meaning that prejudice and discrimination is likely to be a factor for racially differentiated inequalities. For example, racism exists in the workplace, affecting employment levels, pay differences, and overtime opportunities (UNISON, 2016). It exists in sports, as evidenced by Azeem Rafiq's racial harassment experiences in cricketing or the online racial abuse that teenage footballer Bukayo Saka faced after the Euro 2020 Final (Bennett & King, 2021). That same racism contributes to stress levels, which are linked to chronic health conditions in ethnic minority groups, and even extends to care homes (James & Jackman, 2017).

Similar statistics, in fact, exist in the rehabilitation and personal injury field. For example, discrimination in judgements between a 'true' injury versus a 'malingering or exaggerated' illness has been found to be worse for women, immigrants, and Jewish people (Dembe, 1998). Furthermore, if one looks at rehabilitation outcomes in the UK, there is a poorer outlook for ethnic minorities than for the White majority (Fadyl, 2021).

Disadvantage, therefore, arises in many forms and settings. The moment that subjective, social, or political perceptions are involved, the health professional – the likely readership of this book – must recognise their potential to be accessing socially constructed biases, unconscious or otherwise. These can be detrimental to the very people the professional teams are trying to support.

Defining Personal Injury: Claims and the Litigation Process

The medico-legal setting sets the scene for personal injury rehabilitation. *Personal injury* is a legal term used to describe physical or psychological

DOI: 10.4324/9781003309819-10

harm to one's person where fault can be assigned and financial compensation can be sought.

Serious and catastrophic injuries have long-term, life-changing impacts on a client's physical and psychological health and abilities and may include:

- Brain, spinal cord, or orthopaedic injuries;
- Cerebral palsy or birth injuries;
- Amputation; and
- Psychological trauma.

In the UK, according to Barber et al. (2019), 1.4 million people are living with some kind of brain injury. The NHS recorded a compensation spend in 2019 of £100bn for 11,000 patients on clinical negligence claims alone.

What is the 'Medico-Legal Context'?

When someone commences a personal injury claim through the civil courts, the law may award financial compensation. This rehabilitates and restores the individual's functioning, as far as possible, to its likely state before the injury. The financial quantum of the claim must cover:

- Care, rehabilitation therapy support, and equipment;
- Suitable, adapted accommodation, at home or elsewhere;
- Education or workplace adjustments and meaningful leisure or vocational opportunities; and
- Access to the community via suitably adapted vehicles.

The complex task of gathering evidence and supporting the client and family is done by a professional team led by a case manager. This is a social or healthcare professional who assesses, plans, and implements rehabilitation input until the case settles or after settlement.

Kennedy et al. (2015) imply that in determining the extent of injury in the client's personal context, case managers and rehabilitation team members should ensure that clinical decisions are independent of the client's skin colour or cultural background. They should consciously, equally, and without bias advocate for fair treatment in the litigation process and support rehabilitation goals that are right for the client. Yet, the litigation process is built on models of health and well-being that use standards, policies, and procedures of its majority culture. In the UK, the majority culture is White English. In the wake of the Black Lives Matter protests of 2020, the case management industry is only now starting to consider the implications of minority ethnic group experiences in the litigation process. The challenge arises for professional bodies and individual practitioners working in a diverse field to become actively informed, inclusive, and solution-focused for all clients.

Formulation as a Guide for Personal Injury Professionals

This chapter contends that bias should be avoided or minimised, including in the personal injury field, which is driven by a reductionist biomedical model of health and Eurocentric ideas about social, care, therapy, and rehabilitation goals. For effective work with POC and other minority groups, a comprehensive model of personal injury is required to reframe and meet client needs holistically. Ultimately, this minimises distress and improves quality of life within the multi-systemic context. In order to work optimally, personal injury professionals need to develop a therapeutic relationship with the client as well as with the family and colleagues around the client. There is immense value in coordinating all input such that it is integrated in an interdisciplinary way (Larsson-Lund et al., 2022). This contrasts with multidisciplinary working, which Larsson-Lund et al. (2022) purport may not fully maximise outcomes. Psychologists use the method of formulation to invite the client, teams, and family members alike to participate in a holistic and coordinated process of understanding and hypothesising about unmet needs and strategies for meeting them.

Unique Considerations for Formulation When Working with Personal Injury Clients

Given what is known about inequalities and biases in society at large, including within the health, social care, and legal systems, training in person-centred, formulation-based approaches can be of great advantage to any personal injury professional. Cummins et al. (2021) argue that the therapeutic relationship can be a double-edged sword, which facilitates goals but also marginalises clients who are not compliant for various reasons. Client non-compliance can be driven by a number of factors that can make treatment challenging. These can include:

- Psychological trauma;
- Attachment styles;
- Cultural values;
- How language is perceived;
- Team dynamics; and
- Knowing one's own boundaries, professionally and personally.

Psychological Trauma

Psychological trauma typically affects a client's response to decision-making, engagement with rehabilitation, attention to what is being said, recollection of memories, and emotional regulation. A personal injury will likely result in psychological trauma, which requires time to process and a skilled practitioner to notice and work with. Psychological trauma is a significant predictor of injury outcomes, such as returning to work, physical function, and pain (O'Sullivan et al., 2022). Trauma-informed support is therefore vital from professionals working closely with clients. Trauma-informed support, when explored fully, takes into account prenatal as well as past and current traumatic events. This is a crucial step towards understanding clients' (and even their family members') responses to what might seem like a reasonable model of rehabilitation and care. There is therefore a need for personal injury practitioners to become better informed about the socio-political experiences that can influence current and ongoing trauma.

Specifically, racial trauma is caused by exposure to racial or ethnic stereotypes, directly or indirectly. Racial trauma can be difficult for injury clients who identify as POC because, if unresolved, it can be activated by the personal injury experience itself. Despite the 2021 Commission on Race and Ethnic Disparities report findings (Sewell et al., 2021), Statista Research Department (2021) found that 95% of people believe that racism exists in the UK, and 78% believe that racism is more strongly in existence than not. As such, a client who identifies as a POC is likely to have a degree of racial trauma affecting their personal injury experience.

Furthermore, the influence of intergenerational trauma is also of particular interest in this chapter because personal injury clients are typically living within family contexts. Family Systems Theories (Minuchin, 1974; Kerr & Bowen, 1988) purport family as a single emotional unit where the relationships impact on one another. Interestingly, Ford et al. (2015) suggested that due to the cumulative effects of historical and present-day stigma and discrimination, POC are more vulnerable to severe trauma symptoms. This can impede engagement with the professional teams around them and their rehabilitation journey.

Assessing, monitoring, and appropriately addressing the impact of trauma on personal injury clients within their familial and social-political contexts is crucial to lowering anxieties and stress to improve rehabilitation outcomes.

Attachment and Belonging

It is known from attachment theories (e.g., Ainsworth & Bell, 1970) that attachment style is learnt in childhood and determines our relationship patterns in adult life. These attachments are culturally defined, and the beliefs and values that ensue contribute to differences in how different groups of people relate to caregiving practices. While attachment is culturally determined, it refers to a number of interrelated motivations: staying safe, seeking comfort, regulating proximity to the attachment figure, and seeking predictability. It is also linked to a sense of belonging, which can be defined as 'lastingness' or 'continuity' (Baumeister & Leary, 1995). A poorer sense of belonging is linked to psychological distress and poorer well-being (McCallum et al., 2021). Watts (2020) argued that client-professional differences in cultural traditions, attitudes toward illness, and language ability may all affect a client's willingness to participate in rehabilitation.

Bay et al. (2012) found that sense of belonging and interpersonal conflict were important predictors of psychological functioning in mild-to-moderate TBI clients. Relationships with the professional network may therefore be impacted by the attachment style of their client. This suggests that understanding attachment and fostering a sense of belonging can help the professional network to target interventions. For example, it may guide assistance for clients to fit in and feel like an important member of their support and family therapy systems respectively. Douglas (2019) theorised that being misunderstood reduced the sense of belonging for people with TBIs, negatively impacting well-being. The same study found that formal and informal training and education about brain injury significantly improved well-being as a result of clients being better understood.

Cultural Values

Culture is broadly defined as the sum total of ways of living built up by a group of people, which is transmitted from one generation to another. Every community, cultural group, or ethnic group has its own values, beliefs, and ways of living. Cultural values can influence the way others are treated. For example, a client who identifies as being spiritual might prefer listening to prayers and chants as a meaningful occupation over accessing the community for a meal; someone from a more collectivist culture might prefer their family to support them with their personal care rather than a stranger.

Living in a setting where the majority of people do not necessarily share or understand your beliefs or way of living can significantly impact one's quality of life. Bhugra and Becker (2005) talk about cultural bereavement, which is marked by loss of cultural norms, religious customs, and social support systems; adjustment to a new culture; and changes in identity and concept of self. This being a stressful daily experience, it is unsurprising then that mental health and chronic illness rates are increasing in the UK in POC (Bhugra & Jones, 2001).

In personal injury, injury symptoms like pain, sleep, stress, and mood – and therefore rehabilitation – are highly likely to be influenced by feeling culturally bereaved and feeling misunderstood by unsuitable care and rehabilitation models.

Language

Language plays a fundamental role in how individuals perceive themselves and the world they live in. It is undisputed that the words and phrases heard, seen, and said influence a subject's thinking. Language thus constitutes a vital component in the building of a therapeutic relationship with our clients and their families.

When one has experienced an injury, the duty of care that practitioners subscribe to applies from the very moment a referral is read. In the context of bias, trauma, attachment, and the cultural points raised earlier in this chapter, the use of sensitive, respectful, and non-stigmatising language is fundamental. It means thinking carefully about what is said, how it might be received, and whether what is said is helpful to the relationship or not. Medicalised language and terms – such as *scans, bleed, haemorrhage, shock, unstable* – can feel very threatening and unhelpful to clients who have had traumatic histories. In particular, if clients and their families have experienced the trauma of living in war-torn countries or are escaping persecution, language use may be especially critical.

In addition to the kind of language used, it is also essential for professionals to give thought to practical considerations around communicating with clients and colleagues. Examples are the use of language-specific clinicians and culturally-similar professionals as well as knowledge of how the home language describes injury, rehabilitation, impairment, disability, progress, etc. Overlapping with cultural specificity, thoughtfulness also involves absorbing an understanding of the client's and their family's journey to the point they are at now, the flavour of the language as negative or positive, and how much of that is rooted in personal experiences versus how much is defined by home culture.

It becomes clearer why rehabilitation or progress are likely to be less than optimal wherever consideration is not given to the experiences of POC who have migrated from other parts of the globe, to the use of language, and to the many potential sources of miscommunication.

Team Factors

Health professionals who subscribe to holistic approaches to health and well-being, including in the current sense, rehabilitation, will more easily accept that working as a team with a client and their family is going to result in better outcomes. As West and Lyubovnikova (2013) summarised, the evidence in favour of team-based working is the reduced hospitalisations and costs as well as medical error and mortality rates. Sharing ideas about a single client increases effectiveness, innovations, and their implementation in the case. Importantly, service user satisfaction improves with team approaches. Team working also increases the mental well-being of team members, reducing turnover and sickness absences as well as allowing for more effective use of resources.

Creating a therapy team who understand their roles in rehabilitation work requires an understanding of the practicalities of the work (to include home visits, regular liaison with family and professional networks, adequate reporting to the litigation process, etc.). As Madge and Khair

(2000) found, developing clear strategies and coordination across the whole team, inclusive of client and family, is also important in guiding interventions and outcomes. These are preconditions for teams to work optimally, both together and within their own specialisms.

Boundaries

Professional-personal boundaries are common in any profession as a way to define and protect clinicians in their roles, their clients, clients' families, and the organisation for which they work. Boundaries are meant to ensure that relationships between the professionals and the clients and their families do not become personal, even when working on very personal and difficult issues.

Adapting from Hardy (2017), five areas for consideration in medico-legal work are client focus, self-disclosure, dual relationships, working within your competence, and looking after the self. Sound use of reflective supervision and peer support is highly relevant to applying the considerations.

In the medico-legal context, the home setting is hugely influential for setting and maintaining boundaries. Knowing when to remove shoes on entry to a client's home or accepting food offered by a family member or recognising client gender roles from their upbringing and using this understanding helps shape appropriate, meaningful activities. Such thinking requires those who place the client's interests at the forefront of their work to revisit boundaries. They will be informed by values, living patterns, and belief systems.

It is not practical or pragmatic to challenge every potential instance of crossed boundaries in a client's words or actions. The key is to understand the relevance of the proposition and to undertake an ongoing dynamic risk assessment of such situations, intervening where strictly necessary.

A Theoretical Conceptualisation for Personal Injury Professionals: The Personal Injury Formulation and Intervention Model (PIFIM)

The challenge of maximising rehabilitation in a home setting with a team around the client has been reviewed, whilst addressing inequalities in healthcare to minimise distress and unmet needs. To date, there has been no known model for working multi-systemically with personal injury clients, making the challenge harder.

However, the literature reviewed in this chapter clarifies a range of essential components for working well with personal injury clients. Using a multi-systemic structure inspired by models like the Newcastle approach (James, 2017), together with the factors raised earlier, the following new theoretical model is proposed for working with TBI clients, their families, and care teams in a litigation context.

This chapter introduces the Personal Injury Formulation and Intervention Model (PIFIM) (Figure 7.1), an original model that aims to minimise client distress with the team around the client within a legal context. As highlighted, mediators of distress for those experiencing a personal injury can be broken down into several factors, and each informs this formulation and intervention model for rehabilitation work. In addition, we acknowledge a number of psychotherapeutic skills that are required to work competently and in a psychologically safe way with personal injury clients, their families, and the professionals around them. Indeed, some professionals in the field may already be using to some extent the techniques and ideas already raised in this chapter.

In terms of understanding PIFIM, client distress must be first understood as communication by the client themselves, although it is also likely to be reported on and contributed to by family, case management, legal professionals, therapy teams, and care staff. As with any formulation-based approach, all informants in the model proposed are encouraged to share their ideas about what the client needs should distress be noticed. In Figure 7.1, this idea is represented by the 'family', 'legal', 'clinical', and 'care team' perspective labels outside of the circle. Their perspectives can be brought together to contain the ideas, thoughts, observations, and information about the client.

Each informant is invited by the lead clinician to contribute to discussions. Their specialist lenses on the client are brought together to form the parameters of current knowledge and understanding of the client. At this stage, no limits are set on the extent of the information base, nor are hypotheses made. This data gathering exercise is simply used as starting point, an evolving framework based only on what is known today. Through careful and practised interviewing techniques, patterns and connections can be made between specialisms, and the client story begins to form.

The information gathered can be grouped into care plans, client factors, and environmental categories. These three chief categories are applied to help structure the ideas generated by the team around the client. No assumptions are made about which specialists can or cannot add to each category, because it is expected that there would be overlaps between different roles. In order to identify the best-fit client story, attempts must be made to minimise the dynamic risks inherent to power and specialism.

Client factors represent aspects of the internal world of the client, as reported, observed, or assessed by themselves or those around them. Possible domains include life story, personality, pain, sleep, and fatigue levels. If these internal features are triggered negatively in any way, the client may respond in a distressed way. Understanding the degree

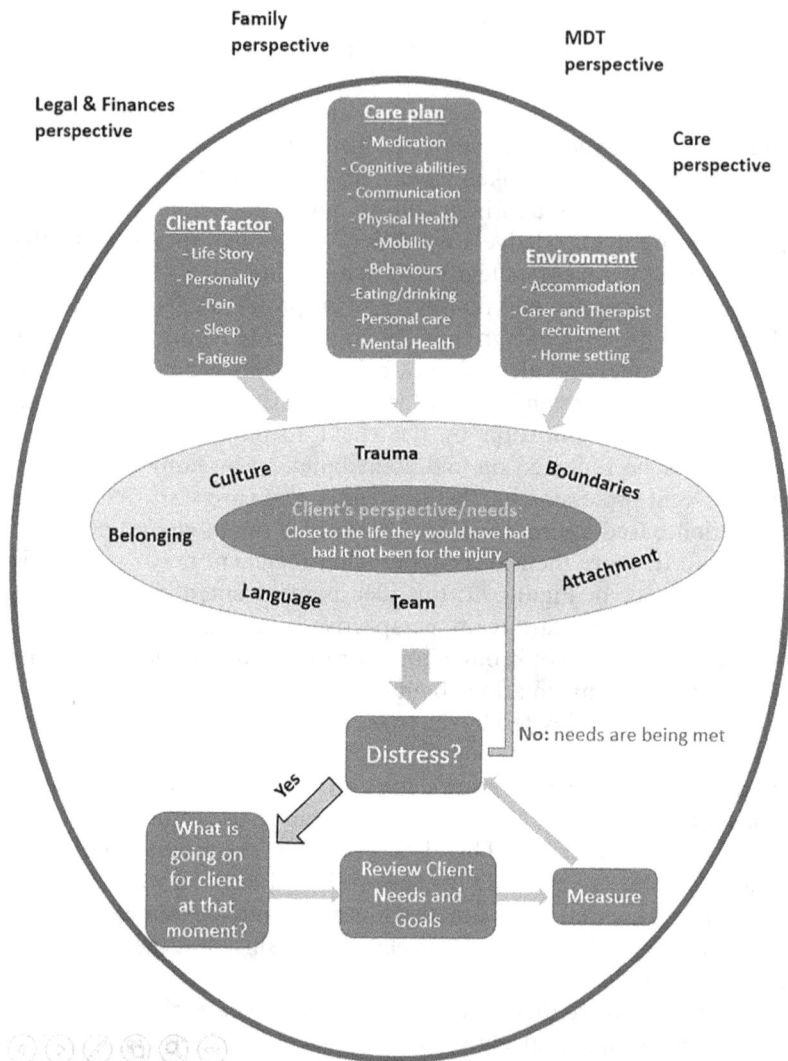

Figure 7.1 The Personal Injury Formulation and Intervention Model (PIFIM): A Multi-Systemic Formulation Guiding Independent Clinicians to Work Interactively as a Team around the Client within the Medico-Legal Context to Maximize Rehabilitation Outcomes

to which these features are taken into account or triggered in the implementation of the care plan can be immensely helpful. It can improve understanding of how the client is perceived, communicated with, and managed, with the aim of improving quality of life and stabilising how the client presents.

The life story is often an excellent way to learn about a client's background extending beyond their present circumstances, which reminds us of the life they might have had prior to their life-changing injury. Their disappointments, drives, motivations, challenges, aspirations, and achievements all form who the client is and how they might subsequently behave. This, of course, becomes an indicator of possible distress that they feel when their needs are not being met. Noticing what is meaningful to a client or how a client relates to their experiences provides a great insight into how they see themselves and others. POC may have a narrative that can be difficult to sit with as a professional; however, once uncovered, it can offer some depth and insight into possible suffering and psychological pain. The extent and severity of pain or discomfort will, of course, vary, but acknowledging it will actively help to bridge a gap and form helpful bonds.

The care plan category refers to the practical guidance around the client's care from a biopsychosocial stance, usually designed for the care team. A care plan will already be in place: they are legal documents that serve to understand the specific client and implement ways to meet their needs under different domains of personal care, health, and functioning. These domains include washing, eating, dressing, toileting, medication, cognitive ability, communications, physical health, mobility, mental health, and risk. Care plan data can be absorbed into the information base and shared with the widest possible range of specialists. Such dissemination supports all parties' understanding of the client's daily routines. It can also point up the challenges that the routines may create for the client, their family, and care teams. 'Meeting needs' can be understood in terms of the way some routines are administered. In the context of PIFIM, those producing the plans must make them as culturally sensitive and individually tailored to the wishes of the client and their family as possible.

The environmental category is focused more on the practical or environmental features which are long-term or core aspects of the client's personal injury journey. These are often difficult factors to rectify quickly, due to them often being beyond the control of members of the widest team or family members. Factors may include suitability of accommodation, professional team recruitment, and the home setting. If there are challenges or disruptions in any of these areas, they will impact on the meeting of the client's needs. Distress is likely to be observed, typically in more parties than the client alone. For example, if accommodation is overcrowded due to extended family living together, this can be inhibiting for the professional team trying to implement their skills. Equally, a client and their family might live in suitably adapted accommodation but recruiting culturally appropriate carers may be problematic. The resulting lack of consistency in the client's routine, the strain on care team members when working with families in the same space, and the family's anxieties all impact the litigation process, therapy goals, and case management relationships.

These three strands feed into the client's needs, as represented in Figure 7.1 at the very centre of the diagram. The notion of living a life as close as possible to the life they would have led had it not been for the injury is defined in terms of overarching aims. Living is, of course, multi-faceted, but here the client and their team are encouraged by the lead clinician to highlight two or three wider aims. Such aims might range from being able to attend school safely to being able to play with one's children or increasing independence in personal-care routines. These are not necessarily specific or measurable per se, but they are an agreed statement for the client and team to focus their input towards. From these aims, more measurable goals can be generated to guide each clinician or carer.

The lead clinician can plan for two to three overarching aims and goals for the team to work on.

Case Study 1: Using PIFIM with a Black Sundanese Adolescent and His Family in a Case Management Assessment

The impact of 14-year-old Client O's near total hypoxic ischaemic brain injury meant that school was poorly attended due to anxiety. The case manager used the model as part of an immediate needs assessment to understand that his anxieties were related to falling due to his hearing loss and hemiplegia. These were heightened by a series of health appointments related to planned surgery in a few months, which his whole family was preoccupied by. It was also challenging for his parents to contain the pressures of their son's rehabilitation goals when the litigation timetable was busy. In addition, his mother, his main caregiver, experienced a complicated labour, which she described as traumatic because the non-Sudanese midwife seemed to ignore her distressed cries for help despite tending to other women. This made it harder for her to trust professionals, which manifested as tearfulness and anger at times. The parents stated a preference for a care team that could represent their Sudanese cuisines and language. This was key as their son liked Sudanese foods and preferred to speak Arabic; therefore, members of the family's community were formally made carers. With PIFIM, the case management team was able to understand the client's distress in terms of an overwhelmed family system that needed support in order to minimise the anxiety exhibited by Client O. Key recommendations for the whole team, driven by PIFIM's mediating factors, included: (a) offering trauma and culture training to amplify the family's needs while also meeting the necessary care standards; (b) holding supervision and team meetings to support appropriate boundary setting between the mother and carers to ensure safe working; (c) communicating to the team around the client the legal timetable so input could be adjusted accordingly; (d) basing all formal meetings on

PIFIM to document improvement and share changes; (e) providing psychological support to help parents respond helpfully to their son; and (f) encouraging joined-up discussions and work across the clinicians, which was reflected in clinicians' update reports.

The agreed overarching goals must then be mediated by underlying process features, such as trauma, culture, belonging, attachment, team working, language, and boundaries, which need to be considered as part of the input. These mediating factors have a dynamic value, as they tend to be expressed interpersonally. This is where the team require skilful support in order to understand life patterns that might exist for the client and how they might play out in their relationships.

Supervision, reflective practice, and self-care carry important roles in negotiating how to navigate client needs within the relationship. This is an important space for professional teams around the client and family to address possible biases. It is in this space that one's openness to racial and traumatic factors can influence the trajectory of the relationship and the alliance that is built. In some ways, it can be argued that this is where the real work happens.

In terms of treatment planning and support, the proposed process for managing client needs can be expressed as being able to observe, hypothesise, review goals, and measure input in order to learn what minimises client distress

Figure 7.1 also proposes an intervention process, as denoted by the lower cycle in the diagram. It suggests a whole-team approach to reduce the distress experienced by the client and to ultimately meet client needs. When information-sharing opportunities are utilised well, there can be more openness to discussing the mediating factors. The process to minimise client distress and meet needs – otherwise termed the intervention or goal phase – can then be progressive and fruitful.

Case Study 2: How to Use PIFIM in Psychology Treatment Work with an Adult Brain Injury Client

Client M, a 35-year-old divorced woman, acquired a moderate brain injury following clinical negligence in minor surgery she underwent as a young adult. She was at risk of her care breaking down and the therapy team disengaging with her. This would have compromised her litigation claim and potentially rendered her much less likely to achieve her goals. She had a complicated family background growing up in China, where her family largely still were. Client M's family would request financial support, which she was not happy about, yet she was fearful of being perceived as selfish. Meeting her family's needs was an important value to her. She struggled to maintain relationships – personal and professional – and feared being lonely should her family disown her; her insight resulted in bouts of low mood and anger. The professional teams felt stuck and concerned about her emotional well-being and risk. PIFIM was used by the treating psychologist to develop the insight Client M had about herself and her life experiences. This allowed the team to develop goals, unpick risks, and support her in accessing aid from her social and professional networks. Training for the care and therapy teams was also provided to understand how relationships could be perceived and how to offer support to Client M, which increased her sense of belonging. Culture-sensitive, formulation-led team meetings resulted in greater understanding of Client M's past and injury-related traumas. This formulation allowed the team to monitor her financial risk in a way that felt safe to Client M. Client M's case settled with her living a life less fearful of family pressure and with a range of personal and carer relationships she was able to sustain with positive goal outcomes.

The intervention circuit offers an opportunity to monitor the information being shared by the team around the client. This is likely to be the care team in a catastrophic injury case, although the therapy team will also contribute here. However, the family around the client will be able to share their experience of client distress with in-situ observations.

If distress is being expressed, the lead clinician will be required to revisit the aims and goals with the team to understand what is happening. This is a difficult task and requires the person to hold many perspectives, narratives, and ideas in mind. Of course, it is possible that an answer remains unclear, so a trial-and-improvement approach might be needed. Care plans, client factors, and environmental issues may need to be refreshed. In addition, the mediating factors may need exploring to unpick where the difficulty might be. Good communication, supervision, training, team meetings, and observations can be used to achieve further clarity here. Goals might need adjusting as a result of revisiting the mediating factors, the outcomes of which must be measured.

If the amendments to the intervention cycle work, then any new understanding can feed back into the formulation part of the model to modify and improve the understanding of the client. If distress remains, the process can be repeated until the client's needs are met. Having a tool that all parties, including the client, can contribute to and that guides the team together towards the agreed goals in a coordinated and client-centred way is the definition of successful rehabilitation.

Conclusion

This chapter has offered a framework to conceptualise the challenges of working with ethnic minority injury clients on rehabilitation programmes. The aim is to minimise client distress and improve quality of life by offering a process that explicitly brings into focus ethnic and racial experiences and differences. Using a psychological formulation-based approach that takes into account the multiple systems around the client allows a coherent and authentic story to be co-created and shared. Maximising rehabilitation outcomes is the ultimate goal of any client, family, and personal injury professional. It is also the right of all clients regardless of their ethnic minority status.

References

Ainsworth, M. D. S., & Bell, S. M. (1970). Attachment, Exploration, and Separation: Illustrated by the Behavior of One-Year-Olds in a Strange Situation. *Child Development, 41*(1), 49–67.

Barber, S., Beard, J., Woodhouse, J., Sutherland, N., Harker, R., Long, R., Kennedy, S., & Powell, T. (2019). *Acquired brain injury.* Commonslibrary.parliament.uk.

Baumeister, R. F., & Leary, M. R. (1995). The need to belong: Desire for interpersonal attachments as a fundamental human motivation. *Psychological Bulletin, 117*(3), 497–529.

Bay, E. H., Blow, A. J., & Yan, X. (2012). Interpersonal relatedness and psychological functioning following traumatic brain injury: Implications for marital and family therapists. *Journal of Marital and Family Therapy, 38*(3), 556–567.

Bennett, M., & King, C. (2021). Taking the knee, mental health, and racism in sport. *The Lancet Psychiatry, 8*(10), 861–862.

Bhugra, D., & Becker, M. A. (2005). Migration, cultural bereavement and cultural identity. *World psychiatry: Official journal of the World Psychiatric Association (WPA), 4*(1), 18–24.

Bhugra, D., & Jones, P. (2001). Migration and mental illness. *Advances in psychiatric treatment, 7*(3), 216–222.

Cummins, C., Payne, D., & Kayes, N. M. (2021). Governing neurorehabilitation. *Disability and Rehabilitation, 44*(17), 4921–4928. DOI: 10.1080/09638288. 2021.1918771.

Dembe, A. E. (1998). The medical detection of simulated occupational injuries: a historical and social analysis. *International Journal of Health Services, 28*(2), 227–239.

Douglas, J. (2019). Loss of friendship following traumatic brain injury: A model grounded in the experience of adults with severe injury. *Neuropsychological Rehabilitation, 30*(7), 1277–1302.

Fadyl, J. K. (2021). How can societal culture and values influence health and rehabilitation outcomes? *Expert Review of Pharmacoeconomics & Outcomes Research, 21*(1), 5–8.

Ford, B. Q., Dmitrieva, J. O., Heller, D., Chentsova-Dutton, Y., Grossmann, I., Tamir, M., Uchida, Y., Koopmann-Holm, B., Floerke, V. A., Uhrig, M., Bokhan, T., & Mauss, I. B. (2015). Culture shapes whether the pursuit of happiness predicts higher or lower well-being. *Journal of Experimental Psychology: General, 144*(6), 1053–1062.

Hardy, R. (2017, June 19). *Top tips on managing professional boundaries in social work.* Community Care. https://www.communitycare.co.uk/2017/06/19/ top-tips-managing-professional-boundaries-social-work.

James, I. A. (2017). The Newcastle model. In I. A. James & L. Jackman, *Understanding behaviour in dementia that challenges* (2nd ed., pp. 148–167). Jessica Kingsley Publishers.

James, I. A., & Jackman, L. (2017). *Understanding behaviour in dementia that challenges.* Jessica Kingsley Publishers.

Kennedy, P., Kilvert, A., & Hasson, L. (2015). Ethnicity and rehabilitation outcomes: The needs assessment checklist. *Spinal Cord, 53*(5), 334–339.

Kerr, M. E., & Bowen, M. (1988). *Family evaluation: An approach based on Bowen theory.* W. W. Norton & Co.

Larsson-Lund, M., Pettersson, A., & Strandberg, T. (2022). Team-based rehabilitation after traumatic brain injury: A qualitative synthesis of evidence of experiences of the rehabilitation process. *Journal of Rehabilitation Medicine, 54,* 1409. DOI: 10.2340/jrm.v53.1409.

Madge, S., & Khair, K. (2000). Multidisciplinary teams in the United Kingdom: Problems and solutions. *Journal of Pediatric Nursing, 15*(2), 131–134.

McCallum, S. M., Calear, A. L., Cherbuin, N., Farrer, L. M., Gulliver, A., Shou, Y., Dawel, A., & Batterham, P. J. (2021). Associations of loneliness, belongingness and health behaviors with psychological distress and wellbeing during COVID-19. *Journal of Affective Disorders Reports, 6,* 100214. DOI: 10.1016/j.jadr.2021.100214.

Minuchin, S. (1974). *Families & family therapy.* Harvard University Press.

O'Sullivan, O., Neale, J., & Mistlin, A. (2022). Rehabilitation After Trauma. In P. Lax (Ed.), *Textbook of Acute Trauma Care* (pp. 819–827). Springer. DOI: 10.1007/978-3-030-83628-3_43.

Sewell, T., Aderin-Pocock, M., Chughtai, A., Fraser, K., Khalid, N., Moyo, D., Muroki, M., Oliver, M., Shah, Samir., Olulode, K., & Cluff, B. (2021, April 28). *Commission on Race and Ethnic Disparities: The Report.* https://www.gov.uk/government/publications/the-report-of-the-commission-on-race-and-ethnic-disparities.

Statista Research Department. (2021, March 29). *To what extent do you think racism is present in UK society today?* https://www.statista.com/statistics/1123242/opinion-on-racism-in-uk-society.

UNISON. (2016). *Guidance for UNISON branches: Challenging racism in the workplace.* https://www.unison.org.uk/content/uploads/2016/11/24073.pdf.

Watts, F. A. (2020, April 11). *Cultural Humility in the Context of Traumatic Brain Injury.* http://www.biact.org/assets/uploads/files/Conference/2020%20handouts/Powerpoints%202020/Cultural%20Humility%20-%20Fatima%20Watt.pdf.

West, K., Greenland, K., & van Laar, C. (2021). Implicit racism, colour blindness, and narrow definitions of discrimination: Why some White people prefer 'All Lives Matter' to 'Black Lives Matter'. *British Journal of Social Psychology, 60*(4), 1136–1153.

West, M. A., & Lyubovnikova, J. (2013). Illusions of team working in health care. *Journal of Health Organization and Management, 27*(1), 134–142.

8 Racial Microaggressions in Neurorehabilitation

Ndidi Boakye and Sue Copstick

Introduction

Racial microaggressions are described as brief and commonplace daily verbal, behavioural, or environmental indignities, whether intentional or unintentional, that communicate hostile, derogatory, or negative racial slights and insults toward people of colour (Sue et al., 2007). For the purposes of this chapter, the terms *people of colour, racialised minorities*, or *minoritised ethnic groups* will be used to describe people of the global majority who do not identify as White. Microaggressions are often described as an unconscious process and, as such, perpetrators of microaggressions can be unaware that they engage in such communication when they interact with members of minoritised ethnic groups. Consequently, if microaggressions are addressed, perpetrators will find plausible alternative explanations to deny of the microaggression. Sue et al. (2007) found that the majority of interracial encounters are prone to microaggressions, which appear in three forms: microassault, microinsult, and microinvalidation.

Microassault is described as an explicit racial derogation characterised primarily by a verbal or nonverbal attack meant to hurt the intended victim through name-calling, avoidant behaviour, or purposeful discriminatory actions (Sue at al., 2007) – for example, referring to someone as 'coloured' or 'Oriental', using racial epithets, discouraging interracial interactions, or deliberately serving or addressing a White patron before someone of colour. Microassaults are most like what has been called 'old fashioned' racism conducted on an individual level (Sue at al., 2007). They are most likely to be conscious and deliberate, although they are generally expressed in limited 'private' situations (micro) that allow the perpetrator some degree of anonymity. In other words, people are likely to hold notions of minority inferiority privately and will only display them publicly when they (a) lose control or (b) feel relatively safe to engage in a microassault (Sue at al., 2007).

Microinsults are characterized by communications that convey rudeness and insensitivity and demean a person's racial heritage or identity. Microinsults represent subtle snubs, frequently unknown to the perpetrator, that clearly convey a hidden insulting message to the

DOI: 10.4324/9781003309819-11

recipient of colour (Sue at al., 2007) – for example, statements such as 'your hair is so interesting/cool' and 'you are so articulate', or the proposing of certain people for opportunities but not others.

Microinvalidations are characterized by communications that exclude, negate, or nullify the psychological thoughts, feelings, or experiential reality of a person of colour – for example, saying 'Oh well, she would feel like that wouldn't she, these x people just can't cope with the job'.

It is important to note that the term *micro* does not equate to the proportion of harm experienced by those on the receiving end of the microaggression. Micro refers to the fact that these experiences take place at the micro level, i.e., everyday interpersonal interactions.

Microaggression in Health Care Systems

Microaggressions are commonly experienced in the NHS – for example, patients report poor access to services or staff report numerous experiences of being 'side lined' when it comes to promotion, discrimination from colleagues and patients, and being excluded from career opportunities (Toft & Franklin, 2020; Kalra, Abel, & Esmail, 2009). One doctor said,

> It can be easy to forget that it's your right to work in an environment that is free from discrimination or marginalisation. Unlike the guidelines available to us when managing a deteriorating patient, tackling microaggressions is something we are forced to learn implicitly, through our interactions with patients and colleagues. Whether it be from a patient inquiring if you are intending to go 'back to where you came from' after training or a consultant attempting a joke about 'you people'.
>
> (Rimmer, 2020)

The same doctor stated,

> Unfortunately, the burden of tackling microaggressions in the workplace falls on those they are directed against. It's everyone's responsibility, however, to create a workplace culture that is both inclusive and nurturing to all. This occurs through careful consideration of our words, silences, actions, and inactions. Therefore, we all have a role in reflecting on how we can use the privileges we have to educate ourselves on challenging microaggressions and removing them from the workplace altogether.
>
> (Rimmer, 2020)

There is evidence that microaggression can do harm. Freeman and Stuart (2018) found that migrant nurses experienced racial microaggression from patients and colleagues through racial preferences and bullying. These microaggressions had a negative impact on their well-being, causing low mood and depression in some instances (Freeman & Stuart, 2018).

Williams (2019) also found that microaggressions are associated with stress (Torres et al., 2010), anxiety (Banks et al., 2006; Blume et al., 2012), depression (Huynh, 2012; Nadal et al., 2014), symptoms of post-traumatic stress disorder (Williams, Printz, & DeLapp, 2018), low self-esteem (Nadal et al., 2014; Thai et al., 2017), substance and alcohol use (Blume et al., 2012; Gerrard et al., 2012), severe psychological distress (Banks et al., 2006; Hurd et al., 2014), reduced self-efficacy (Forrest-Bank & Jenson, 2015), and suicide (Hollingsworth et al., 2017; O'Keefe et al., 2015).

Williams (2020) states that experiencing a microaggression signals a dangerous environment, resulting in corresponding psychological and physiological stress responses (e.g., Clark et al., 1999). Reactions following experiences of microaggressions may include confusion, anger, anxiety, helplessness, hopelessness, frustration, paranoia, and fear (Williams, 2020). In addition to stress, this may lead to dysfunctional coping strategies, such as denial, withdrawal, and in some cases substance abuse (Williams, 2020). Microaggressions are so commonplace, they are now being understood as a form of chronic stress which may contribute to health problems, such as hypertension and impaired immune response (Berger & Sarnyai, 2015; Clark et al., 1999). Evidence of the impact of microaggressions on health is still emerging.

Microaggressions also cause harm in other ways, such as contributing to barriers to treatment (e.g., Walls et al., 2015). Experiencing microaggressions carried out by clinicians can undermine the therapeutic relationship among patients of colour, who may in turn avoid care (Freeman & Stewart, 2018). This can impact engagement with services (Owen et al., 2014), which directly affects treatment outcomes.

Microaggression in Neurorehabilitation

Loya and Uomoto (2015) argued that the dynamics in the relationship between staff and patients had not been given adequate attention. They highlighted that the counselling and psychotherapy literature was replete with evidence of the therapeutic relationship being a predictor of good clinical outcomes. Therefore, any potential sources of strain or disruption required addressing in a timely manner. This necessitates clinicians to understand aspects of their own behaviours and ways of interacting with patients that may cause fissures in the relationship, particularly in cross-cultural therapy dyads. To date, there has been little discussion about this in the field of neurorehabilitation (Loya & Uomoto, 2015) or neuropsychology. Furthermore, there is little professional guidance on how staff working in neurorehabilitation settings can be supported to understand how cultural factors impact rehabilitation processes and outcomes.

One way in which staff can negatively impact the therapeutic relationship is by engaging in racial and ethnic microaggressions towards their patients. As Sue (2005) stated, helping professionals are part of the general public and, as such, are not immune from the sociocultural developmental processes that shape racial and ethnic prejudices, some of which impact how patients are viewed and treated. This in turn can enforce the broader negative societal attitudes and disrupt treatment goals.

The following cases are examples of the different types of microaggressions that might transpire in neurorehabilitation settings.

Case Vignette One

The team are discussing a young Muslim male who has had a stroke. He cannot walk and has difficulties with impulse control. He is 21 years old, presents with challenging behaviour, he is reported to 'hold the gaze of female staff leaving them feeling uncomfortable, and asks them out on dates'. The team have had difficulty engaging with the family. There is only one sister who can communicate in English, and she is keen that her brother returns to the family home. The team (largely White females) report that he is not engaging in rehabilitation, but they are unable to evidence this. They report that the sister is the only 'sensible' member of the family, and they want to inform her that her brother isn't engaging in services and should be discharged home. The patient is in his first two weeks of rehabilitation. The service offers a specialist 12-week MDT rehabilitation program. There is no further support in the patient's home borough.

Case Vignette Two

An Indian, female, first-year trainee psychologist is in a team meeting waiting for the family of a patient to join. One of the staff members – a White male OT –says to the trainee, who is observing the session, 'Do you know what type of brain injury this patient has? You probably don't know the answer but give it a try'. He proceeds to ask her about the patient's brain injury. The trainee uncomfortably answers, and the OT expresses his surprise that she is correct. He shouts a loud 'well done' whilst laughing, not noticing the uncomfortable smiles from other members of the team in the meeting.

Case Vignette Three

A 50-year-old Black Jamaican woman on holiday in the UK is admitted to the ward following a traumatic brain injury. She is paraplegic. On her first morning on the ward, the nursing team report her as 'aggressive and displaying challenging behaviour'. They state that they 'couldn't understand her' and she was 'loud and impatient' when asked to repeat herself. On exploration with the nursing manager, the patient reported that she had requested twice if she could have a shower but was ignored by the staff and told she had to have breakfast.

The case examples above highlight the complex ways in which microaggressions play themselves out in neurorehabilitation settings. They all raise questions about their potential impact on the rehabilitation process and quality of care. In the first and third case studies, the question is how does the team's treatment of the patient (and family) impact on the relationship with the service? Could it limit treatment effectiveness or engagement in the rehabilitation process? Furthermore, could it impact the family's relationship to help? Could the team's behaviour become the norm and shape how the service interacts with patients and families from minoritised backgrounds?

The type of microaggressions for each case are highlighted below (Table 8.1).

Addressing Microaggressions

In order to address microaggressions when examining the case examples above, clinicians should ask themselves: How do you feel when reading this vignette? What do you notice happening to you? What thoughts/images

Table 8.1 Microaggressions Unpacked

Case	Type of Microaggression	Microaggression unpicked
Vignette 1	Micro-invalidation	The largely white female team *report that the sister is the only "sensible" member of the family*, The fact that she is the *only* member of the family that *speaks English* affords her the title of *'sensible'* underlying prejudice views that the non-English speaking members of the family are not sensible.
Vignette 2	Micro-invalidation	The white OT derogatively stated that "*you probably don't know the answer*, but give it a try", he also expressed his surprise that the Indian trainee clinical psychologist is correct. and shouts a loud "*well done*". Underlying the OT's behaviour are unconscious prejudiced ideas about the level of intelligence the trainee has. The level of comfort in communicating this view also highlights the privilege the OT operates in; he is not challenged by his colleagues nor does he self-monitor his behaviour. Both highlight the power Whiteness and being male affords him.
Vignette 3	Microinsult	The nursing team view the 50-year-old Black Jamaican woman as *loud and aggressive* in keeping with prejudiced ideas of black people. There is little discussion about the patient's dignity and if that was the reason she asked to be returned to her room. Stereotypical assumptions and pathologisation of racially minoritised individuals can led to an increase in negative judgements, labelling and shaping harming narratives. It can also shape the trajectory of their clinical treatment leading to iatrogenic harm.
		The interpretation of her accent causing a breakdown in communication is also a microinsult underlying prejudiced ideas of what constitute normal accents or accepted ways of speaking.

come to mind? What are the contexts of prejudice, power, and privilege that make this situation possible? Based on your personality, style, and position, how would you address this situation? What barriers do you perceive to speaking up or taking action?

Training and reflective practice are key in helping clinicians navigate the interactions in which microaggressions take place. There are no clear or straightforward answers (Loya & Uomoto, 2015). This work is still very much in its infancy in the UK and is multi-layered. For patients (and families) with multiple intersecting identities, microaggressions can occur at many levels (e.g., ethnicity, gender, disability, sexuality, nationality, and much more). Loya and Uomoto (2015) highlight that in neurorehabilitation services it may be assumed that individuals with brain injury, stroke, and other neurological disorders are in the 'majority' culture because their disability is acquired. However, they may also experience other forms of microaggression, such as ableism, e.g., staff speaking freely in front of someone with poor memory because 'they won't remember anyway'.

For minoritised ethnic groups living with brain injury and grappling with disability, they face multiple challenges, such as increased health inequalities and being twice as likely to be living in poverty as compared to those without disabilities (Allwood & Bell, 2020: van Kessel et al., 2022). The consequences of living in poverty include low academic success, food insecurity, increased odds of living in an unsafe area, poor access to health care resulting in decreased physical health, increased stress and depression, and, if employed, a greater chance of working in jobs associated with higher risk for injury and death (Tansey et al., 2016).

Telhan et al. (2020) stressed the need for clinicians to understand the link between systemic trauma and health, as without this acknowledgement the conditions we treat may ultimately remain refractory in the absence of remedies to the structural issues that underlie and perpetuate them. They suggested that the trauma-informed care model may be a useful starting point. The trauma-informed care model is predicated on the notion that trauma is defined not only as interpersonal maltreatment but also as structural and sociohistorical violence, which can underlie medical dysfunction. For example, in the case of a patient with brain injury, a broad trauma-informed approach (Figure 8.1) would rigorously inquire about the structural circumstances, such as racism, economic inequality, and access disparities, leading to brain injury, such as stroke, as well as downstream barriers that might impede rehabilitation outcomes. Telhan et al. (2020) stressed that these contexts rarely enter meaningfully into the awareness of rehabilitation practitioners. If they did, such awareness may inform our care for individuals and communities. Going forward, neurorehabilitation practitioners may benefit from the adoption of the trauma-informed principles to optimise the care and treatment outcomes of the neurological population. This is particularly pertinent when designing new services and condition-specific pathways.

Safety	•Throughtout the organisation, staff and the people they serve feel physically and psychologically safe
Trustworth-iness and transparency	• Organisational operations and decisions are conducted with transparency and the goal of building and maintaining trust among staff, clients and families of service users
• Peer Support and mutual self-help	•These are key to the organisation and service delivery, key for building trust, establishing safety and empowerment
• Collabora-tion and mutality	•Recognising that healing happens in relationships and in the meaningful sharing of power and decision making. Everyone has a role to play in a trauma informed approach. You do not have to be a therapist to be therapeutic
• Empower-ment, voice and choice	•The staff, service users and family members' experience of choice is strengthened. There is a recognition of everyone's individuality and building on what resources everyone has to offer rather than responding to perceived deficits
• Cultural historical and gender issues	•The organisation moves past cultural stereotypes and biases and offers culturally responsive services and recognises and addresses historical trauma

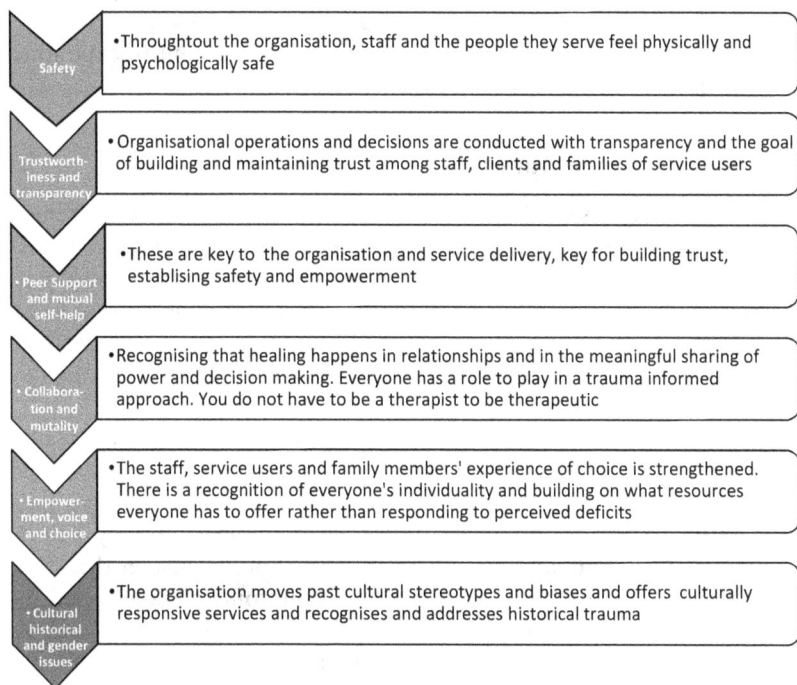

Figure 8.1 Trauma-Informed Principles
(Harris & Fallot, 2001)

For professionals, Sue (2010) suggests the following:

1. Actively get acquainted with people who are different from you in terms of beliefs, culture, or other qualities. We tend to stick with what we know, what is familiar to us. A lot of microaggression is around ignorance and lack of knowledge;
2. Be aware of your defence mechanisms at play when someone points out you may have biases verging on prejudice;
3. Call out discrimination and bias yourself – silence can perpetuate the cycle.
4. Follow the three As:
   • **Activate inclusion**: Facilitate an educational, clinical, or social event where staff can spend time just sharing their perspectives. This enables an understanding of different thoughts and perspectives, which increases shared experience and therefore support acceptance and involvement with others.
   • **Ask about diversity**: Find out how your colleagues from different backgrounds experience their work, as feeling marginalised can

result in withdrawal. As neuropsychologists, we can support colleagues and patients in expressing their perspectives.

- **Accept personal responsibility**: Make a commitment to expand to accommodate a new view or world view.

Further Actions to be Taken

1. More research is needed on our patients' and colleagues' experiences of microaggression. Currently, our case studies do not feature the effects of social behaviours, such as prejudice and microaggression, as barriers to recovery and rehabilitation. A better understanding can increase the quality of our care and clinical outcomes. We have ways of assessing microaggression and gender/race/religious bias, and our journals should encourage this consideration in studies.
2. In our clinical outcome measures we do not consider feelings of isolation as a proxy for whether people feel they are (or are not) included or accepted. So many people with a brain injury feel less than they were before the brain injury. Acceptance and inclusion may well be key to adjustment, and outcome measures should consider this.
3. Further attendance is required to the symptoms of race-based injury that occurs between patients and helping professions, such as race-based trauma manifesting as mistrust or anxiety. This should be accounted for in the formulation and psychological treatment.
4. We should promote job matching and working with people from a variety of cultures and characteristics as a key part of our professional development, including appropriate training, support, and supervision. This will likely improve our practice as it forces us to consider wider factors in our clinical formulations.
5. We should promote regular reflective practices and openly discuss the impact of culture on our work. This includes the consideration of Whiteness.
6. We have an awareness of the impact of microaggression on our colleagues, patients, and their families or friends. We need to identify, validate, and manage microaggression where appropriate. Policies with guidance covering the aforementioned points can be a useful starting point in supporting staff to address microaggressions.
7. We should ensure that our practice, our supervisees, and those we manage reflect an awareness of microaggressions, their impact, and how to support those on the receiving end of them.

Conclusion

Neurorehabilitation is not shielded from the experience of microaggressions, as clinicians' views reflect those of the public. It is therefore not uncommon to see it manifest in day-to-day work. However, the research suggests that microaggressions are harmful for patients, their families, and staff. Training and ongoing reflection are key to developing recognition and awareness of the impact of microaggressions on the therapeutic relationship and the patient journey. Policies and guidance that encourage self-reflection and open dialogue can lead to a more inclusive rehabilitation environment with better outcomes for clinicians, staff teams, patients, and their families.

References

Allwood, L., & Bell, A. (2020, 18 June). Covid-19: Understanding inequalities in mental health during the pandemic. *Centre for Mental Health*.

Banks, K. H., Kohn-Wood, L. P., & Spencer, M. (2006). An examination of the African American experience of everyday discrimination and symptoms of psychological distress. *Community Mental Health Journal*, *42*(6), 555–570. DOI: 10.3109/10253890.2014.989204.

Berger, M., & Sarnyai, Z. (2015). 'More than skin deep': stress neurobiology and mental health consequences of racial discrimination. *Stress*, *18*(1), 1–10. DOI: 10.3109/10253890.2014.989204.

Blume, A. W., Lovato, L. V., Thyken, B. N., & Denny, N. (2012). The relationship of microaggressions with alcohol use and anxiety among ethnic minority college students in a historically White institution. *Cultural diversity and ethnic minority psychology*, *18*(1), 45–54. DOI: 10.1037/a0025457.

Clark, R., Anderson, N. B., Clark, V. R., & Williams, D. R. (1999). Racism as a stressor for African Americans: A biopsychosocial model. *American psychologist*, *54*(10), 805. DOI: 10.1037/0003–066X.54.10.805.

Forrest-Bank, S. S., & Jenson, J. M. (2015). The relationship among childhood risk and protective factors, racial microaggression and ethnic identity, and academic self-efficacy and antisocial behavior in young adulthood. *Children and youth services review*, *50*, 64–74. DOI: 10.1016/j.childyouth.2015.01.005.

Freeman, L., & Stewart, H. (2018). Microaggressions in clinical medicine. *Kennedy Institute of Ethics Journal*, *28*(4), 411–449. DOI: 10.1353/ken.2018.0024.

Gerrard, M., Stock, M. L., Roberts, M. E., Gibbons, F. X., O'Hara, R. E., Weng, C. Y., & Wills, T. A. (2012). Coping with racial discrimination: The role of substance use. *Psychology of Addictive Behaviors*, *26*(3), 550–560. DOI: 10.1037/a0027711.

Harris, M. E., & Fallot, R. D. (2001). *Using trauma theory to design service systems*. Jossey-Bass/Wiley.

Hollingsworth, D. W., Cole, A. B., O'Keefe, V. M., Tucker, R. P., Story, C. R., & Wingate, L. R. (2017). Experiencing racial microaggressions influences suicide ideation through perceived burdensomeness in African Americans. *Journal of Counseling Psychology*, *64*(1), 104–111. DOI: 10.1037/cou0000177.

Hurd, N. M., Varner, F. A., Caldwell, C. H., & Zimmerman, M. A. (2014). Does perceived racial discrimination predict changes in psychological distress and substance use over time?: An examination among Black emerging adults. *Developmental psychology*, *50*(7), 1910–1918. DOI: 10.1037/a0036438.

Huynh, V. W. (2012). Ethnic microaggressions and the depressive and somatic symptoms of Latino and Asian American adolescents. *Journal of youth and adolescence*, *41*(7), 831–846. DOI: 10.1007/s10964-012-9756-9.

Kalra, V. S., Abel, P. and Esmail, A. (2009). Developing leadership interventions for Black and minority ethnic staff: A case study of the National Health Service (NHS) in the UK. *Journal of Health Organization and Management, 23*(1), 103–118. DOI: 10.1108/14777260910942588.

Loya, F., & Uomoto, J. M. (2015). Racial and Ethnic Microaggressions in the Neurorehabilitation Setting. In J. M. Uomoto (Ed.), *Multicultural Neurorehabilitation: Clinical Principals for Rehabilitation Professionals* (pp. 251–272). Springer. DOI: 10.1891/9780826115287.0010.

Nadal, K. L., Wong, Y., Griffin, K. E., Davidoff, K., & Sriken, J. (2014). The adverse impact of racial microaggressions on college students' self-esteem. *Journal of college student development, 55*(5), 461–474. DOI: 10.1353/csd.2014.0051.

O'Keefe, V. M., Wingate, L. R., Cole, A. B., Hollingsworth, D. W., & Tucker, R. P. (2015). Seemingly harmless racial communications are not so harmless: Racial microaggressions lead to suicidal ideation by way of depression symptoms. *Suicide and Life-Threatening Behavior, 45*(5), 567–576. DOI: 10.1111/sltb.12150.

Owen, J., Tao, K. W., Imel, Z. E., Wampold, B. E., & Rodolfa, E. (2014). Addressing racial and ethnic microaggressions in therapy. *Professional Psychology: Research and Practice, 45*(4), 283–290.

Rimmer, A. (2020). How can I tackle microaggressions in the workplace? *BMJ, 368*, m690. DOI: 10.1136/bmj.m690.

Sue, D. W. (2005). *Multicultural social work practice.* John Wiley & Sons.

Sue, D. W. (Ed.). (2010). *Microaggressions and marginality: Manifestation, dynamics, and impact.* John Wiley & Sons.

Sue, D. W., Capodilupo, C. M., Torino, G. C., Bucceri, J. M., Holder, A., Nadal, K. L., & Esquilin, M. (2007). Racial microaggressions in everyday life: Implications for clinical practice. *American psychologist, 62*(4), 271–286.

Tansey, T. N., Dutta, A., Kundu, M., & Chan, F. (2016). From admiration of the problem to action: Addressing the limited success in vocational rehabilitation of persons from diverse racial and cultural backgrounds. *Journal of Vocational Rehabilitation, 45*(2), 117–119.

Telhan, R., McNeil, K. M., Lipscomb-Hudson, A. R., Guobadia, E. L., & Landry, M. D. (2020). Reckoning with racial trauma in rehabilitation medicine. *Archives of Physical Medicine and Rehabilitation, 101*(10), 1842–1844.

Thai, C. J., Lyons, H. Z., Lee, M. R., & Iwasaki, M. (2017). Microaggressions and self-esteem in emerging Asian American adults: The moderating role of racial socialization. *Asian American Journal of Psychology, 8*(2), 83–93. DOI: 10.1037/aap0000079.

Toft, A., & Franklin, A. (Eds.). (2020). *Young, disabled and LGBT+: Voices, identities and intersections.* Routledge.

Torres, L., Driscoll, M. W., & Burrow, A. L. (2010). Racial microaggressions and psychological functioning among highly achieving African-Americans: A mixed-methods approach. *Journal of Social and Clinical Psychology, 29*(10), 1074–1099. DOI: 10.1521/jscp.2010.29.10.1074.

Van Kessel, R., O'Nuallain, E., Weir, E., Wong, B. L. H., Anderson, M., Baron-Cohen, S., & Mossialos, E. (2022). Digital health paradox: International policy perspectives to address increased health inequalities for people living with disabilities. *Journal of medical Internet research, 24*(2), e33819.

Walls, M. L., Gonzalez, J., Gladney, T., & Onello, E. (2015). Unconscious biases: Racial microaggressions in American Indian health care. *The*

Journal of the American Board of Family Medicine, 28(2), 231–239. DOI: 10.3122/jabfm.2015.02.140194.

Williams, M. T. (2019). Adverse racial climates in academia: Conceptualization, interventions, and call to action. *New Ideas in Psychology, 55,* 58–67. DOI: 10.1016/j.newideapsych.2019.05.002.

Williams, M. T. (2020). Microaggressions: Clarification, evidence, and impact. *Perspectives on Psychological Science, 15*(1), 3–26. DOI: 10.1177/1745691619827499.

Williams, M. T., Printz, D. M. B., & DeLapp, R. C. T. (2018). Assessing racial trauma with the Trauma Symptoms of Discrimination Scale. *Psychology of Violence, 8*(6), 735–747. DOI: 10.1037/vio0000212.

9 Harnessing Technology to Level the Playing Field

A Route to More Efficient and Accessible Services in Rehabilitation

Penny Trayner

> The thing my service needed didn't exist, so I made it.
> Penny Trayner, paediatric clinical neuropsychologist, DJ,
> healthcare technology entrepreneur

Introduction

In many ways technology is the ultimate leveller. By using technology, individuals, including staff and patients accessing services, can gain access to knowledge and skills that they might not otherwise have, thereby breaking down barriers and levelling the playing field. When the right technology is used in the correct way, it can be transformational.

Our personal lives have become increasingly managed and organised by technology, and there is ever-evolving crossover into our professional lives in terms of how and when technology is deployed. This chapter will discuss two examples from my own experience of using technology to address clinical and administrative problems in rehabilitation. My own background is purely clinical. It is a result of being a user of technology within my personal life that I have been open to opportunities where technology can be used to enhance my clinical practice. This chapter details firstly my journey from fledgling DJ to designing a programme that uses DJing as a vehicle for delivering rehabilitation, and secondly my experiences in developing Goal Manager®, a project that arose entirely organically through trying to find a solution to a problem.

My Journey to DJing for Rehabilitation

Being a DJ and a psychologist is essentially the same job – the ultimate goal of both is to make people happier.

In 2019, I had the opportunity to attend an intensive 'zero to hero' course through the 'Lisa Lashes School of Music', a first-of-its-kind model developed by the first and only woman to feature in *DJ Magazine*'s top ten DJs in the world ('Lisa Lashes', 2022). In three months the course took me from

DOI: 10.4324/9781003309819-12

absolute beginner to a paid, professional DJ. It was an astonishing new chapter in my life and one for which I am very grateful, particularly as it sparked the idea of using DJing as a vehicle for delivering rehabilitation.

A complex rehabilitation programme involving multiple therapies can take up a lot of time. Motivation to engage can wane over time, particularly where clients are trying to juggle multiple life demands as well as trying to meet all the demands of their therapy programme. As a paediatric neuro-psychologist, I am responsible for overseeing children's rehabilitation from a clinical perspective, ensuring that we are measuring progress and linking our work clearly back to the functional needs of the individual. I also must deliver a programme that is relevant, meaningful, and motivating.

Brain injury can affect people from all backgrounds, ethnicities, and incomes. My service covers children living in council estates in the most deprived areas of the UK as well as children attending some of the top private schools in the country, however the majority live in areas of high deprivation. Approximately 17.5% of my service users are from Black or other non-White backgrounds. Brain injury survivors are already marginalised due to the impact of their injuries, regardless of ethnicity or social background. However, due to the location of my service, nearly all of our service users come from deprived areas. Therefore, all our work-flows, interventions, and technology innovations are specifically aimed at being as accessible and cost-effective as possible.

As soon as I began my own training it was immediately obvious that there is a huge potential for core rehabilitation skills to be targeted through DJing, both practically in the skills themselves and in the planning and organising around it. I set out to design a DJing rehabilitation programme, which was piloted as part of a four-day, non-residential summer camp, 'Brain Bootcamp', in 2019. Camp participants received psychoeducation and training in cognitive skills in the mornings, then they had the opportunity for real-world application of their knowledge through learning to DJ in the afternoons. The DJing element of the pro-gramme was delivered by DJ Mark One, an international award-winning DJ, lecturer, and national assessor for accredited graded music examina-tions in DJing. Mark has been a professional DJ since 1991, playing in clubs, festivals, and arenas as well as on TV and radio. Since 2001 Mark has specialised in bespoke tuition programmes in DJing and focuses on teaching versatility to students across a range of abilities, including mix-ing ability, the understanding of music, the hardware and software, and helping students to habituate to clubs and other musical environments.

How Can DJing Assist in Rehabilitation and What is the Role of Technology?

When many of us picture DJing, we envision expensive and complex equipment and the need to lug around huge crates of vinyl records. This may be an activity clearly inaccessible to many; however, DJing has long been recognised as a very skilled and desirable art form (Smart et al., 2019). This latter point is important as research suggests that, following an acquired brain injury, many survivors can experience a loss of social identity and support (Muldoon et al., 2018). Finding opportunities for survivors to develop positive self-esteem and connect with others is our constant mission as rehabilitation providers. Many people have positive memories of nights out and events they have attended, which have been facilitated by music. Finding a way for people to be a part of that has a long-standing history of being successful within rehabilitation, where the use of music therapy in rehabilitation is now well established (Magee et al., 2017).

Modern DJing involves digital equipment which can be automated to suit the needs of the individual. There are so many settings and adjustments that can be put in place to make DJing accessible to almost anyone. DJ equipment can be set up to adjust the degree of motor involvement, and preprogramming can reduce both the cognitive and motor demands. Students can become competent more quickly and get the reward and gratification of being able to mix their own music, also meaning they are able to practice immediately and build their skill more quickly.

Core skills targeted by DJing include:

Motor and Coordination

Controlling DJ equipment, mixing, and scratching require motor skills and coordination. Psychomotor coordination and processing speed are also targeted by the coordination of auditory input with cue timing to start up tracks at different points.

Visual Processing

Visual processing is required to access the visual displays on the software and/or digital media player, to search through the music collection, and to view the information about individual tracks, including their unique waveforms (Smart et al., 2019).

Attention and Concentration

Auditory attention skills are targeted through listening to songs and tracking the progress of the music to locate the right mix points as well as through identifying 'space' in the music to add things such as sound effects. Again, this can be made more accessible according to the needs of the DJ. Modern DJing uses software to organise and play out the music, where cue points can be pre-programmed in advance (Smart et al., 2019). During the set, all the DJ has to do is look out for the cue point and then press a button to start the next track. If required, the software can automatically match the beats and even mix one track into the next. This significantly reduces the cognitive demands, meaning that the individual is more likely to have a successful and enjoyable performance.

There are also a lot of simultaneous tasks, which require both divided and attention-switching skills. DJs are required to divide their attention between the track that is currently playing and the upcoming track. DJs also are required to switch between different tasks, for example altering the equaliser (EQ) levels whilst adjusting the volume and starting another track all at the same time. Selective attention skills are also used to pick out particular elements of the music. Sustained attention is required to help DJs keep focused on the task and maintain their attention in order to complete the entire set and to sustain their attentiveness on individual tracks in order to not miss mix points.

Memory

DJs learn about the structure and content of music as well as performance skills. Memory skills are also targeted when organising and compiling playlists and remembering the order of tracks. Working memory skills are targeted by listening to a track and actively counting along with beats and bars at the same time as part of the mixing process.

Executive Functions

Planning and decision-making skills are targeted in the selection of music tracks, the choosing of mix points and the style in which the tracks will be arranged together, and in deciding the overall playlist and atmosphere of the set. Much like composing a concert, playing a set involves arranging the music to take the listeners on a musical journey (Smart et al., 2019). Decision-making skills are targeted through track selection and decisions on how to play out particular tracks. No DJ will ever play the same music exactly in the same way, which means that DJs really have the opportunity to express their own individuality and creativity.

DJing also involves an element of behavioural control in initiating, controlling, and inhibiting behaviour in order to play tracks and mix them together successfully. There is an element of managing the emotional demands of the situation to stay calm in order to execute a good set. As in any activity or performance, things can and will go wrong. There is a real opportunity to use DJing as a safe way to engage in real-world problem-solving, exploring coping skills, and helping develop resiliency to challenge.

Being a successful DJ involves planning, structure, and staying organised, not only concerning the organisation of set lists and tracks within the individual's collection but also diarising lessons and events as well as keeping up to date with practice. This encourages individuals to make use of compensatory strategies, such as diaries, planners, and checklists, to aid them in all aspects of these tasks. DJing provides a meaningful and motivating reason to use these strategies, which is particularly relevant for individuals who may have experienced a significant decrease or entire loss of their previous social life and activities. It can be very hard to find the motivation and drive to engage without a reason to do so.

Confidence and Self-esteem

By harnessing technological advances in DJing, we can help individuals to be successful at it very quickly. In our experience so far, this has brought an enormous sense of positive self-worth and meaning and purpose to individuals' lives. DJing has a popular peer perception. Being able to DJ equips individuals with something they can feel proud of and is a means for them to connect with society at a time when they have potentially lost or changed their previous relationships. For individuals who are no longer able to participate in a sports team or other group activities they enjoyed prior to injury, or for those who are no longer able to participate in the same way, the loss of or change to the social connections that are an integral part of those activities can have a profound effect on mood and motivation. DJing is intrinsically motivating for so many young people and provides a vehicle for social engagement and interaction.

Generalisability

Within the literature for cognitive rehabilitation after acquired brain injury (ABI) in children, there is ongoing debate as to the relative value of restorative (e.g., training discrete cognitive skills) versus compensatory (e.g., environmental optimisation) approaches (Forsyth, 2010; Limond & Leeke, 2005). Whilst individual cases of improvement are reported, there is currently no conclusive evidence for the efficacy of cognitive rehabilitation following an ABI (Limond & Leeke, 2005; Ross, et al., 2011). In terms of retraining cognitive skills (restoration), there is limited, but modest, evidence for the effectiveness of some interventions, mainly with regard to the training of attention skills. However, the generalisability of any gains to everyday functioning has yet to be established (Forsyth, 2010; Ross, et al., 2011). Given that executive functioning skills may be critical in children's use of strategies across all cognitive domains, broadly-focused rehabilitation approaches may be the ideal target for intervention. Such approaches target executive functioning and overall adaptive functioning in everyday tasks. Specific strategies may then be added to target any residual cognitive impairments (Limond &

Leeke, 2005). The aim is to maximise functioning across all domains in order to broaden opportunities for future educational and vocational activity and independence.

A great body of evidence from animal studies has demonstrated that environmental enrichment can have a profound effect on recovery after ABI (Forsyth, 2010). Precisely what constitutes an enriched environment in children and young people is less clear; however, the school and family environment (including family 'coping style') can be a powerful mediator (Forsyth, 2010). School and other educational contexts provide 'rehabilitation' in and of themselves by offering opportunities for peer contact and thus opportunities to practice and model social, emotional, and communication skills. It is essential, therefore, that rehabilitation is ecologically valid and delivered in meaningful contexts (Forsyth, 2010). However, after a catastrophic brain injury it can be hugely challenging for people to find such places in the world.

One of DJ Mark One's favourite quotes is that 'DJing is a gateway' to many other opportunities in life. There are many different roles within the music industry to which DJing can open the door. Mark's story of how he became a professional DJ is truly inspirational. He learned first as a teenager in his bedroom, at a time when he did not even own any turntables. Instead, he used an old drum kit and mixer and copied the DJs he watched on music videos (Smart et al., 2019). From this start, he went on to become an internationally renowned DJ. DJing gave Mark a focus and purpose to his life. It can do the same for brain injury survivors, giving a meaningful and motivating focus for their rehabilitation.

Results from the Brain Bootcamp Pilot Study

The pilot of the DJing programme, delivered as part of the 2019 Brain Bootcamp, was hugely successful. In our evaluation, the young people who attended showed an increase of resilience, optimism, self-efficacy, trust, and comfort as well as a reduction in vulnerability (Trayner & Dowson, 2020). By the end of the week, everyone in the group was able to DJ and produced a 20-minute mix as a showcase of their achievement. They had also learned to use and apply a variety of compensatory skills, and they had had the opportunity to socialise and interact with their peers. For the majority of the young people who attended, this was the first time that they had had the opportunity to interact with someone with an acquired brain injury. The value of this social contact and peer learning cannot be overstated and was remarked upon by both the group participants and their parents as one of the most positive outcomes of the programme. There were reports of increased engagement with their wider rehabilitation, greater integration with peers, and positive feedback from parents as well as the participating young people.

Case Study – Ollie

Ollie is the mixed-race child of a single mother who is in receipt of universal credit and lives in a town that is within the top 2% of most deprived areas in the UK. Ollie was 11 years old at the time of the Brain Bootcamp and had an acquired brain injury as a result of meningitis infection shortly after birth. He attended a specialist school as a result of significant language, learning, and behavioural difficulties and had previously been diagnosed with attention deficit hyperactivity disorder (ADHD). Ollie also presented with aggressive behaviour, oppositional and defiant behaviour, and rule-breaking behaviour. The characteristics of his brain injury limited his insight and awareness, meaning he was susceptible to influence from aberrant peers within his neighbourhood. He had to be very closely monitored by his family and was generally not able to go out alone into the community as a result of his vulnerability.

Prior to the Brain Bootcamp, Ollie and his family had received approximately 12 months of individualised neuropsychological rehabilitation and behavioural management support; however, his difficulties with attention, concentration, and behaviour, in particular, were persistent and present at the start of the programme.

Everyone who had previously worked with Ollie expressed surprise at the remarkable change in his presentation and behaviour, both at and following the Brain Bootcamp. Ollie enthusiastically took on board the learning and engaged with all the strategies. He expressed himself eloquently in the discussions in the morning and made some really deep, meaningful, and valid points. He was kind and thoughtful, and he said some very endearing things to the rest of the group, including his message to himself that he should 'never jump out of the light' as his learning from the week. Ollie was extremely keen to continue with DJ sessions, and it was clear how this activity has been beneficial to him, not only in terms of his concentration and attention skills but also in terms of giving him the opportunity to use his memory and his planning and organising skills. His progress had given him a real sense of pride, accomplishment, and achievement. He also demonstrated a lot of natural aptitude for the music. Since the Brain Bootcamp, Ollie has continued with DJing lessons, has performed at a festival, has recently passed Grade I music exams in DJing, and is now studying for higher Grades. He has continued to maintain the gains that were noted at Brain Bootcamp. Importantly, DJing gave Ollie back a sense of his social identity, as he now had a skill that made him 'cool' to peers and increased his social currency.

Case Study – Lily

Lily is the child of White, working-class parents and lives in an area which is within the top 5% of the most deprived areas of the UK. Lily was 12 years old at the time of the Brain Bootcamp. She had been injured in a road traffic accident two years prior, when she was struck by a car and sustained a severe traumatic brain injury. Lily presented with significant cognitive and behavioural difficulties, including memory problems, learning problems, difficulties with attention and concentration, and executive function difficulties. She was subsequently diagnosed with ADHD and presented with significant neuropsychiatric difficulties, including a diagnosis of major depression and personality change as a result of her acquired brain injury and self-injurious behaviours. Lily attended a challenging mainstream high school that had recently been placed into special measures. This meant that the support on offer to Lily from school was somewhat fragmented and inconsistent. At the time of the Brain Bootcamp, Lily's behaviour was very erratic, and she was struggling to get on with her family and peers at school, with a lot of issues involving interactions on social media.

Although Lily was a delight in terms of her bright and cheerful manner, she struggled with impulsivity and disinhibition throughout the Camp, which worsened as she became more tired across the week. It was noted that this did cause some frustration amongst the group; however, it was managed in a safe and supportive manner. This gave important information for how Lily is perceived by others in her everyday life, which then informed intervention planning. Despite her struggles, Lily showed a remarkable memory for all the information covered. It was wonderful to see her demonstrate her knowledge with confidence, also adding in her own interpretations. It was noted that as soon as she stepped up to the decks, she would become much calmer and entirely focused on the task. She also made use of all the suggestions and coping strategies from the cognitive skills workshops and was really annoyed at herself one day when she had forgotten the notebook where she had carefully documented her learning from the week.

Lily was very keen to continue DJing and, after a break of over a year, she resumed DJing lessons and showed an incredible amount of retention of the knowledge and skills, even after this time. Lily wants to use DJing as an opportunity to help her to feel calmer and deal with difficult emotions and as a way of connecting socially with others.

DJing/Brain Bootcamp Summary

Research suggests that being part of a social group with others also affected by similar difficulties plays a key role in promoting health and well-being. It also reduces feelings of disability (Muldoon et al., 2019). Unfortunately, for many ABI survivors such opportunities are rare. Following on from the Brain Bootcamp pilot, DJ Mark One and I developed a structured DJing for rehabilitation programme, BPM Rehab ('Brains Powered by Music'), which is now available to adults and young people throughout the UK. Lessons are delivered either face-to-face or virtually so that they are accessible to almost everyone, wherever they may be. This means that BPM is accessed by a wide social and ethnic demographic, with representation across the board in terms of equality and diversity. Participants can and do bring their own interests and identity to their music and performance. The programme can lead to accredited qualifications in music as well as opportunities to develop other skills, such as music production and presentation skills. The aim is to not only provide a meaningful and purposeful rehabilitation activity, but also to create a pathway to increased social contact and engagement with everyday life.

The price of DJ equipment varies, but entry-level equipment now has all the features of larger models used in clubs. A controller (all-in-one decks and mixer) can be purchased for under £150, and music can be streamed from a smartphone or tablet. The cost to attend the BPM course is often met from rehabilitation funds, where these are available to individuals, as it constitutes part of their rehabilitation activity. We have also established a social enterprise to provide subsidised equipment and lessons to individuals who may otherwise struggle with access. We are also building capacity within the community through 'trainer training' in schools and rehabilitation settings.

Having an activity which gives value, purpose, and meaning can be really useful in forming a focus for the direction of rehabilitation, which is of value to the individual. Working towards something meaningful ensures that the reasons for all the rehabilitation activities are clear. Rehabilitation goals that are valued and personal increase participation in rehabilitation (Wade, 2009).

Goal planning is a core activity of rehabilitation, and the following section will explore how technology helped solve an administrative challenge in rehabilitation goal planning by automating the underpinning processes and workflow, freeing more time to focus on real-world, valued, clinical activities with service users.

Technology Can be Used in Healthcare to Leverage More Time

The field of medical technology concerns the development of scientific and technological solutions to address health problems or issues (Tulchinsky & Varavikova, 2014). This definition encompasses an array of technologies and approaches, including those used directly in the delivery of healthcare, such as diagnostic procedures or medical and assistive devices. There are also technologies that help organise services and perform administrative duties to help healthcare professionals carry out their work more effectively and efficiently, reducing the burden on them so that they can direct their efforts towards clinical practice.

Unfortunately, whilst healthcare services continue to be stretched, there is no shortage of clinical need. This led me to consider what other aspects of my role could be supported and improved through the application of technology to streamline and make my processes more efficient to free up my time to focus on the actual clinical work.

Most clinicians are familiar with the use of electronic patient record (EPR) systems. The UK's National Health Service (NHS) began the transition to the use of EPR in the early 2000s. This involved multiple systems across different services, most of which did not communicate with each other (Department of Health and Social Care et al., 2020). The great vision of all services being linked up and a smooth electronic pathway seamlessly connecting the acute hospital setting to community services was not realised. Technology frustration is rife amongst healthcare professionals. A survey of NHS clinicians conducted by the UK government found the greatest frustrations identified included: slow, unreliable hardware; taking too long to log in; patient records not being accessible when needed; difficulties getting new technology commissioned; outdated software; difficulties building new digital services on existing platforms; difficulties in communicating with colleagues; and the use of obsolete technologies, such as faxes and pagers (Department of Health and Social Care et al., 2020). The onset and rapid development of smartphone technology gave us the power to use these tools to organise our home lives in a way that was not possible for many of us at work. It also took a long time before these home systems could securely communicate with work systems, meaning people had to have multiple devices as well as multiple logins.

It has been 20 years since the first EPR systems appeared in the UK, and they are now a commonplace feature in almost all services. EPR systems provide benefits in terms of the sharing of data within individual services, data security and privacy, communication between colleagues, and the use of such systems to schedule appointments, particularly where patients can self-schedule; however, many of these systems have problems, are clunky to use, and do not entirely fit the needs of services (Department of Health and Social Care et al., 2020). The onset of the COVID-19 pandemic meant that digital transformation was accelerated, as in-person contact was restricted due to regulations aimed at reducing the spread and transmission of the virus. This necessitated the increased use of remote appointments and virtual clinical intervention. Services turned to these technologies and found ways to ensure that patients continued to receive clinical input. Many of these changes have been adopted on a more permanent basis, with an international survey of neuropsychologists (Hammers et al., 2020) suggesting that 90% of respondents intend to continue using telemedicine for clinical interviews, 59% for testing, 88% for feedback, and 70% for intervention.

Whilst digital growth has revolutionised services, it is essential that the technologies underpinning those services are fit for use. It is an ideal time for services to conduct internal audits of their procedures and identify areas where technology may improve the efficiency of service delivery. This was an issue that I was already considering within my own service prior to the COVID-19 pandemic.

As the clinical lead for the rehabilitation teams with whom I work, I am responsible for overseeing the goals of rehabilitation, ensuring that the multidisciplinary team's activities are working effectively towards these goals, and making sure that progress is tracked and reported in a timely, clear, and useful manner. To do this effectively was a time-consuming and increasingly infeasible task. Workflow tools automating administrative procedures in healthcare settings were recognised as having potential for cost-saving in administrative expenses over two decades ago (Latamore, 1999). However, when I searched for a digital solution for managing rehabilitation goal setting, it simply did not exist.

Over the past few years, I have discussed goal-setting procedures with countless service providers from all over the world, all of whom share the same need but also lack a solution. Previously, my own practice consisted of tracking client goals using text documents and spreadsheets to organise the data. This involved compiling information from different members of the team. The data was frequently recorded in multiple different formats, and each therapist had different ways of reporting and tracking goals. Manually compiling this data in a manner that communicated it clearly and concisely took up a huge amount of time, and the process of doing so really lost the nuance of goal setting as an activity. We became so weighed down in the administrative requirements of the task that there was less time to focus on the content of the goals themselves.

I decided to set about designing my own solution.

Goal Manager®, which was developed in late 2018 as a programme to use in-house within my service, was designed to organise and report our goal data and clinical activity. The aim was to improve efficiency by streamlining, simplifying, and automating the time-consuming stages involved in rehabilitation goal setting. However, it quickly became apparent that the application had the potential to be of benefit much more widely (Trayner, 2020). Working very closely with a software developer, I set about building a platform to be fit for use for a variety of teams working with any health condition concerned with setting client goals, setting actions towards achieving these, and tracking progress toward attainment. Goal Manager® features the entire International Classification of Functioning, Disability, and Health (World Health Organization, 2001), as I wanted to ensure that this was a solution that would be applicable across the range of healthcare so that people would be able to access a familiar platform, using a common language, wherever they worked.

Goal Manager® quickly became invaluable in helping us to organise our clinical activity and that of the teams with whom we work. We have been able to increase the number of people we are able to see, as we are not spending as much time on administration. Problems are more readily identified and progress can be more easily tracked, also providing vital evidence for continuing funding of treatment.

As a result of my experience in developing Goal Manager®, many other ideas have been sparked in terms of further areas where we can innovate and improve. As clinicians we take total accountability for our patients' care, and this should include the underpinning infrastructure which provides this patient care.

Helping Services to Adopt New Technologies

Innovation and a choice of technology are, of course, extremely important; however, usability and interoperability are arguably the most important factors (Department of Health and Social Care et al., 2020). Social media platforms, apps, and websites all have a consistency and continuity about their structures and organisation, which allows us to navigate these platforms more readily and easily (Krug, 2014). By taking these same principles and applying them to healthcare applications, we can have access to technology that works as seamlessly as it does in our home lives.

A key factor in the success of adoption of new technology in services is providing the right amount of support, training, and leadership for changes to take place effectively (Galen Data, 2022). Usability testing has identified that, just as at home, we will often get started with something without thoroughly reading the manual. Individuals will often use technologies as best they can, without any training whatsoever (Krug, 2014). People expect software to be simple and intuitive to use, and the challenge is for clinicians who are not familiar with building software platforms to design with this knowledge in mind. Training and support should be tailored to the needs of each individual, depending on their level of familiarity and comfort in using technology, and such training should be ongoing as required.

Undoubtedly, a lack of resources and funds to implement technology is a core issue (Department of Health and Social Care et al., 2020; Pearl, 2014). It is therefore important that clinicians who are familiar with the everyday experience of services are directly involved in the design of such technologies, so that they are more likely to be utilised. Once there are demonstrable benefits, it is much easier to make business cases for additional funding for further investment and development.

Organisations such as the Academic Health Science Networks (AHSNs), founded in 2013, have been instrumental in supporting small and medium enterprises (SMEs) in bringing their technology to the public sector. Within the private sector, the onset of social networking and virtual collaboration means that getting innovations to the market is a much easier process. If your product works, you can get it promoted and used in a way that is much easier than ever before. However, it is perhaps unrealistic that busy clinicians, already burdened with extensive clinical responsibilities, have the time to do this and, therefore, clinical, academic, and business partnerships are essential.

Clinicians need to be empowered to put forward our own clinical needs and ideas for technological solutions and then work in partnership with technology companies to develop these. Otherwise, clinicians will continue to endure technology solutions that are a poor fit and fail to meet the needs of the end users. My call to action is for industry procurement leads to be looking beyond big technology companies and seek the direct advice of clinicians and service users. They should be the drivers of innovation and work in partnership with the expertise offered by experienced technology companies.

Advice for Implementing New Technologies in Services

- When looking to implement a new technology, start small. Work with a small number of cases initially or identify a small number of clinicians to get used to using the new system, and then build up from there.
- Tailor training to the needs of the individual. Work with your team's strengths, preferences, and needs. Find out how comfortable, confident, and competent staff feel in the use of technology in general and use this information to help guide the structure of training.
- Provide ongoing training. All of us have the experience of logging on to a previously used programme or platform that has been upgraded, and suddenly we find ourselves unable to navigate it. That feeling of insecurity can be mitigated by providing the appropriate amount of training and ensuring it is ongoing.
- If you are to be a champion for technology within your own service, then you too need to be confident and competent. Ensure you get your own training and address any challenges. These difficulties are likely to be experienced by at least some members of your team.
- Be radical. If you have an idea, you can make it happen. Clinical academic partnerships with business are key to this working. There are many private-, public-, and charitable-sector technology schemes and funding opportunities. It is an ideal time for clinicians to take their rightful role in the development of technological advances in healthcare. If you are working in a clinical service and find that you need something that does not exist, it is likely that many others like you around the country and the world will be experiencing exactly the same challenge.

Summary and Conclusions

I am a huge proponent of the use of technology. However, solutions need to be fit for purpose and add clinical value, either through direct therapeutic benefit or by freeing up time and resources by making individuals' jobs and lives easier (Galen Data, 2022). What I have learned from my experience in developing Goal Manager® is that, whilst the processes involved in developing a digital technology can be lengthy, complicated, and costly, they are not insurmountable. However, if clinical services are truly to get the best and fastest benefit from technological advances, it is essential that clinicians have the opportunity to work in partnership with technology companies so that solutions are developed which are fit for purpose. If the private sector gains access to the latest technologies and innovations ahead of National Health Service, this creates inequality, as those accessing private services get the best available tools and technologies. By harnessing technology, we can ensure that all services have a similar level of skill in terms of how they organise and deliver their services. By reducing the unrelenting demands on the public-sector services and releasing some of the time needlessly spent on laborious but necessary procedures and tasks, we increase our chances of making healthcare more equitable for all.

Nevertheless, introducing technology innovations into services is challenging. Clinicians and service users are at different levels of competence and comfort in using technology. It can seem easier to simply carry on with things the way they are rather than introduce a new challenge (Pearl, 2014), particularly where clinicians are already stretched and feeling under pressure from work demands. In a 2020 Health and Care Professions Council (HCPC) consultation on updating the Standards of Proficiency for Practitioner Psychologists, it is proposed that psychologists must be 'able to change their practice as needed to take account of new developments, technologies, and changing contexts' (Health & Care Professions Council, 2020, p. 14). This recognises the inescapable intertwining of technology in the professional lives of psychologists and other healthcare professionals.

Using healthcare technology increases access to the best level of healthcare for the greatest number of individuals by automating processes to improve the accuracy and efficiency of healthcare processes (Galen Data, 2022). Developments in technology also offer increased accessibility by supporting activities which were previously inaccessible and by enabling participation (Aranda-Jan, 2020). Through technology we can make real progress in accessibility even in the absence of an increase in the availability of services or funding. By using technology, we can help all individuals make the best use of the skills they have and learn the best skills they can.

It is important to acknowledge that technology can also create greater inequality due to issues such as geographical location and internet connectivity, literacy and digital skills, which can further limit people who are already marginalised from making full use of technology (Aranda-Jan, 2020). These are ongoing challenges which need to be addressed from an infrastructure perspective in partnership with technology companies. Ultimately, only those who are actually able to access the technology will benefit from using it (Xplor Technologies, 2021).

Similarly, many developers of technologies that may be helpful to others may also be locked out of being able to further their ideas due to inequalities within funding. A study of 2019 investment data by Cornerstone Partners (2021) found that the majority of venture capital funding went to individuals from advantaged socio-economic backgrounds, mainly graduates from prestigious universities, with funding more likely to go to founders who have been to the most exclusive universities. Black and racially minoritised women and non-binary founders were found to be the worst represented. The report rightly concludes that many marginalised groups are precluded from funding at this very early stage.

Research consistently demonstrates disparity in opportunities and outcomes for entrepreneurs in the UK (Cornerstone Partners, 2021). Women from ethnic minority backgrounds are systemically disadvantaged; however, even when controlling for factors such as sector, part-time working, and household income, the disparities persist (British Business Bank, 2020). The 2020 Diversity Beyond Gender report found that women who identified as Black received just 0.02% of investment and South Asian women received 0.8%, in comparison to White women who received 9.2% (Brodnock, 2020). There is not a level playing field for entrepreneurship, and factors such gender, ethnicity, social-economic status, and geographical location create disparity from the outset (British Business Bank, 2020).

Despite the challenges, the mission to implement digital change is a worthy one. At this stage it seems unlikely that we will see such rapid expansion of service provision that we will have sufficient cover to provide the gold-standard services that we all aspire to. A viable solution is to leverage technology to make better use of the time that we have, to look for opportunities where we can simplify, and to speed things up. This will help us to release our time in order to dedicate it to essential, non-administrative clinical activity.

References

Aranda-Jan, C. (2020). *The mobile disability gap report 2020*. GSMA. Retrieved from https://www.gsma.com/mobilefordevelopment/wp-content/uploads/2020/12/GSMA_Mobile-Disability-Gap-Report-2020_32pg_WEB.pdf.

British Business Bank. (2020).*Alone, together: Entrepreneurship and diversity in the UK*. Retrieved from https://www.british-business-bank.co.uk/wp-content/uploads/2020/10/Alone-together-Entrepreneurship-and-diversity-in-the-UK-FINAL.pdf.

Brodnock, E. (2020). *Diversity Beyond Gender: The state of the Nation for diverse entrepreneurs*. Extend Ventures.

Cornerstone Partners. (2021). *The Cornerstone report: Access to venture capital*. Retrievedfromhttps://report.cornerstone-partners.co.uk/wp-content/uploads/2021/04/Cornerstone-Report-2021.pdf.

Department of Health and Social Care, NHS England, & NHS Improvement, NHS Digital. (2020). *Digital transformation in the NHS*. National Audit Office. Retrieved from https://www.nao.org.uk/wp-content/uploads/2019/05/Digital-transformation-in-the-NHS.pdf.

Forsyth, R. J. (2010). Back to the future: Rehabilitation of children after brain injury. *Archives of Disease in Childhood, 95,* 554–559.

Galen Data. (2022). The disadvantages of technology in healthcare. *Galen Data*. Retrieved from https://www.galendata.com/disadvantages-of-technology-in-healthcare.

Hammers, D. B., Stolwyk, R., Harder, L., & Cullum, C. M. (2020). A survey of international clinical teleneuropsychology service provision prior to and in the context of COVID-19. *The Clinical Neuropsychologist, 34*(7–8), 1267–1283.

Health & Care Professions Council. (2020). *Standards of Proficiency: Practitioner Psychologists [DRAFT]*. Retrieved from https://www.hcpc-uk.org/globalassets/consultations/2020/standards-of-proficiency/practitioner-psychologists/practitioner-psychologists---revised-standards-of-proficiency.pdf.

Krug, S. (2014). *Don't make me think, revisited: A common sense approach to web and mobile usability*. New Riders.

Latamore, G. B. (1999). Workflow tools cut costs for high quality care. *Health Management Technology, 20*(4), 32–33.

Limond, J., & Leeke, R. (2005). Practitioner review: Cognitive rehabilitation for children with acquired brain injury. *Journal of Child Psychology & Psychiatry, 46*(4), 339–352.

Lisa Lashes. (2022, January 29). *Wikipedia*. Retrieved from https://en.wikipedia.org/wiki/Lisa_Lashes.

Magee, W. L., Clark, I., Tamplin, J., & Bradt, J. (2017). Music interventions for acquired brain injury. *Cochrane Database of Systematic Reviews, 1*(1), CD006787. DOI: 10.1002/14651858.CD006787.pub3.

Muldoon, O. T., Walsh, R. S., Curtain, M., Crawley, L., & Kinsella, E. L. (2019). Social cure and social curse: Social identity resources and adjustment to acquired brain injury. *European Journal of Social Psychology, 46*(6), 1272–1282. DOI: 10.1002/ejsp.2564.

Pearl, R. (2014, September 11). 5 things preventing technology adoption in health care. *Forbes*. Retrieved from https://www.forbes.com/sites/robertpearl/2014/09/11/5-things-preventing-technology-adoption-in-health-care/?sh=1e360e6b6889.

Ross, K. A., Dorris, L., & McMillan, T. (2011). A systematic review of psychological interventions to alleviate cognitive and psychological problems in children with acquired brain injury. *Developmental Medicine & Child Neurology, 53,* 692–701.

Smart, A., Smart, S., & Dent, T. (2019). *How to DJ: A guide to DJ-ing and electronic music*. Faber Music Limited.

Trayner, P. (2020). Using software technology in neurorehabilitation to facilitate effective, time-efficient goal-setting. *Archives of Physical Medicine and Rehabilitation, 101*(11), E49–E50.

Trayner, P., & Dowson, M. (2020). *Rehabilitation in the real world: An exploration of meaningful community interventions for young people with acquired brain injury* [Poster presentation]. Annual Conference of ACRM, Atlanta, Georgia, USA.

Tulchinsky, T., & Varavikova, V. (2014). Health technology, quality, law and ethics. In T. Tulchinsky & V. Varavikova (Eds.), *The new public health* (3rd ed.) (pp. 771–819). Elsevier Academic Press.

Wade, D. T. (2009). Goal setting in rehabilitation: An overview of what, why and how. *Clinical Rehabilitation, 23*, 291–295.

World Health Organization. (2001). *International classification of functioning, disability and health (ICF)*. World Health Organization.

Xplor Technologies. (2021). Why technology holds the key to widening access in today's world. Retrieved from https://www.xplortechnologies.com/gb/resources/blog/why-technology-holds-key-widening-access-todays-world.

10 Queering Neuropsychology

Rob Agnew

Introduction

In the last five to ten years, there has been an increase in awareness of the existence of LGBTQ+ individuals who have rehabilitation/treatment needs following a neurological event or illness and how these needs may differ from the cisgendered (non-transgendered), heterosexual population. Having reviewed the research in this area, the field of clinical neuropsychology appears to be revealing itself as a considerate and forward-thinking ally of the LGBTQ+ communities. There is a sincere, although modest, effort to explore the complexity in the practice and provision of sensitive and effective rehabilitation.

It is difficult in one chapter to consider the complexity of every LGBTQ+ group for every relevant clinical consideration (indeed, the term itself does not account for most of the communities which it is used to denote). To avoid this problem, this chapter will consider some conceptual issues that might allow any clinician to 'queer' their practice. 'Queering' is a term given to the process of considering a subject from perspectives which corrupt or question the mainstream understanding of that subject. It is derived from queer theory, a field of critical academic enquiry that emerged most notably in the 1990s alongside the work of scholars in gender and feminist theory, such as Judith Butler (1990), and adopts the deliberate reclamation of the homophobic slur 'queer' (previously used to indicate 'something that differed from the norm'). It is hoped that this approach might allow some level of modification at the conceptual level to our practice to increase inclusivity.

In this chapter, I will forego the term 'LGBTQ+' and instead use 'sexual orientation, gender identity, and relationship diverse' (SOGIRD) communities. I hope this will refocus this text on the shared experiences of oppression from a heterocentric, cisgendered society as a consequence of flouting gender norms. This approach also will include, at least by implication, the often unincluded minority-within-minority groups (e.g., kink, pansexual, intersex, non-binary groups, and others). Where individual texts refer to the communities in a different way (e.g., 'LGBT'), I will, for accuracy, default to that written term for that citation. I will

DOI: 10.4324/9781003309819-13

use the contraction 'trans' rather than 'transgender(ed)', as feedback I have had from individuals in the trans community in my lectures is that this term is softer and less medicalised. Finally, this chapter will not include consideration of 'sexuality' as opposed to 'sexual orientation'. The psychosexual ramifications of neurological injury are outside the scope of the socio-political matters of concern to the SOGIRD communities in neurorehabilitation practice described in this chapter.

The World Context for SOGIRD Communities

At the time of writing this chapter, 71 countries criminalise SOGIRD (LGBT+) peoples, with 11 offering the death penalty (Human Dignity Trust, 2022). In Eastern Europe and Russia, government policies passed since 2013 have legitimised and effectively decriminalised the hunting, torture, and murder of LGBTQ+ people (Human Rights Watch, 2018). The UK in 2021 saw the highest levels of LGBTQ+ hate crime since 2015, with a 210% rise in homophobic crime and 322% rise in transphobic crime (Hunte, 2021). As minoritised groups, SOGIRD individuals are acutely aware of the constant 'push and pull' that exists in society and in legislation regarding our rights. These struggles in other countries highlight the fragility of the accomplishments of the SOGRID communities in securing our rights in the UK and are a source of anxiety and concern for our global community. Social media has connected fragmented groups like never before, but the stark reality of the lived experiences of our communities in different parts of the world serves as a reminder that although the world may exist in turbulent layers of tolerance and oppression, it rarely offers full welcoming acceptance to SOGIRD peoples.

In the 21st century, a SOGIRD-aware clinician should consider seriously the impact of mainstream and social media commentary on health and mental health. A recent survey by Stonewall found that 10% of LGBT individuals had experienced online homo/trans-phobic bullying in the month preceding the study (Stonewall, 2017). In mainstream media there is widely disseminated problematic commentary from individuals such as JK Rowling (Petter, 2020) and television presenters like Piers Morgan (Maurice, 2019), who opine in such a way as to cause outrage and distress to SOGIRD individuals. These individuals and political organisations (e.g., The LGB Alliance, Transgender Trend) often claim that they are in support of trans rights and, under the defence of free speech, are publicly pitted against trans individuals, who end up having to defend their existence instead of debating the issue at hand (McLean, 2021).

Where these individuals articulate their position, they succeed in reiterating the arguments of the 1980s and 90s that gay men, bisexuals, and lesbians had some success in overcoming. Now it is trans people who are a threat to children and women, who threaten the fabric of society, and who simply make life choices that they do not have an 'inalienable right' to (Margaret Thatcher's Anti-Gay Speech, 2013). Bisexuals, however, may have a different experience of the media as they are barely acknowledged, a phenomena called 'bi-erasure' (LGBT Foundation, 2020). The fact that a bisexual person may have heterosexual and homosexual sex appears to make irrelevant the full characterisation of their potential sexuality by both cisgendered heterosexual (cis-het) and SOGIRD communities. Furthermore, their experience of society goes unappreciated, undervalued, and unacknowledged.

In the UK Courts there has been some movement towards inclusion and equality for trans people. In 2021, the Keira Bell vs Tavistock and Portman NHS Health Foundation (2020) ruling was overturned in the Court of Appeal (2021). This ruling would have seen transgender youth denied basic human/health rights regarding Gillick competence and self-determination for gender affirming treatment. Some progress was made in 2022 with a UK Government consultation on the proposed banning of conversion therapy for children and adolescents, which is widely regarded by professionals and learned bodies as a harmful and ineffective set of pseudo-scientific procedures that attempt to change sexual orientation (Jowett et al., 2021). However, there was also regression in the proposed self-identification of gender identity changes to the Gender Recognition Act (2004) by the UK Government. This involved the withdrawal of support for lowering the requirements for obtaining a gender recognition certificate, a process trans people can find humiliating and traumatic.

It is important also to consider that trans people who are also from minoritised racial and ethnic groups often experience another layer of discrimination and oppression from within SOGIRD groups. Racism and bigotry exist across society; inhabiting one difference does not make one immune to being discriminatory of another. So too, where intersectionality exists there is an especially heightened level of threat for the SOGIRD individual. The Black transgender community have recently voiced that they are particularly at risk of crime, and this is due to compounded socio-economic factors and gender-identity-based discrimination (Fischer, 2021), but also to a disproportionate level of violence against this group (Human Rights Campaign, 2021). Often SOGIRD individuals cannot access support within their ethnic or religious community for the discrimination they experience based on their race, ethnicity, or religion. This is because there may be discrimination from within that ethnic/racial/ religious demographic group due to the SOGIRD individuals' sexuality or gender identity (Butler et al., 2010). It must also be considered that where multiple aspects of oppression and privilege coexist, they can appear to compound or mask one another. For example, White gay men may experience fewer challenges in employment than gay Black men where there is evidence that both sexuality and race are factors upon which discrimination is based (Drydakis, 2021; Office of National Statistics, 2020).

SOGIRD people are arguably more visible than at any other time in history, and they have succeeded in accessing some rights. However, the increase in overt media aggression towards our trans community is evidence that being louder and more visible makes for an easier target. There is very much a sense of 'two steps forward and one step back'. The clearest most recent example in Western society can be found in the United States. In March 2022, the Floridian Senate gave support to the 'Don't Say Gay' bill, which bans schools from talking about SOGRID issues and originally required schools to report a suspected gay, lesbian, bisexual, or transgendered child to their parents (Florida State Senate, 2022). Analogous to the UK's Section 28 of the Local Government Act (UK Government, 1988), which was regarded to be hugely damaging to SOGIRD communities, this marks a sad regressive step for the United States.

We have more voice, and we are more seen. However, this was no award from an enlightened cis-hetero-centric society. It was hard won, and every day it must be re-won.

Conceptual Challenges for Clinical Neuropsychology

Western psychology has not been a universally benevolent endeavour for all peoples. On the contrary, it is historically politicised and largely responsible for the consolidation of the eugenics movement in the early 20th century (Yakshuko, 2019). This movement informed the ideology of Nazi Germany and the subsequent horrific acts against LGBTQ+ individuals during the Second World War. In America this anti-LGBT philosophy extended into the field of psychoanalysis (Izzard, 2000) and the pathologisation of homosexuality despite Freud's originally progressive position on the matter. This medicalisation resulted in various 'treatments' for issues of sexuality that resulted in the emergence of what are considered conversion therapies (Smith, 2004), which were once regarded to be embedded in good clinical science and have since been strongly evidenced to be ineffective and harmful (Jowett et al., 2020).

As psychometricians and therapists, clinical neuropsychologists should appreciate that many of the assumptions that underpin our current practice can still be traced back to problematic origins, and we should take an irreverent stance towards our claim to knowledge.

(Gender) Essentialism

A core problematic assumption in gender identity and sexuality-sensitive practice is that of essentialism. This is the idea that there exist in some realm, extraneous to ours, 'ideal forms' for that which we can perceive and conceive of. Themselves, these ideal forms/essences are said to be unalterable, but they are thought to predetermine what a thing shall become (Grayling, 2021). The common example given is that of a perfect circle. Ten artists may draw ten freehand circles. All may be different in microscopic ways, but all attempt to approximate the ideal form/essence of the perfect circle. All artists have an understanding of something that is a perfect circle, an ideal that exists somewhere, but that does not necessarily exist in the realm which is available to our senses. Essentialist assumptions underpin a great deal of the Western philosophical, epistemological, and psychological reasoning that has emerged over the last two-and-a-half thousand years. For example, one can argue that personality, cognitive modularity, emotions, memory are all predicated on the idea that there is a perimeter around each concept – each is encapsulated and represents some type of 'prototypical blueprint', which when corrupted leads to dysfunction.

The concept of gender-essentialism (the idea of there being a prototypical 'man' and 'woman' essence that biology attempts to realise in each conception) has been thoroughly addressed, and there exist more parsimonious and convincing arguments that relieve us of the need for this understanding of gender and sex (De Beauvoir, 2021; Butler, 1990). The contribution of psychology and neuroscience to the evidence for this is also being deconstructed (Hyde et al., 2019; Rippon, 2020). The tendency towards essentialist processing itself has been established as a cognitive bias that emerges early in infancy (Gelman, 2005). It also emerges in the context of an environment of stimulation and social interaction, which allows the development of subsequent, cognitive functions.

Whilst the tendency towards essentialist thinking may be innate, the bias it causes us to manifest in our reasoning is one that we must control for. The effect of essentialist accounts of difference, i.e., race, is understood as often being connected to prejudice (Mandalaywala, 2017), and where our clinical reasoning relies on essentialist theories we should be wary of inadvertently discriminating against our clients.

Othering and Minoritisation

'Othering' is a term first formally outlined by Spivak (1985) in a paper relating to the postcolonial construction of India in discourse and history. It refers to the process by which a group is distanced from the mainstream or dominant group and held at bay by multiple social mechanisms. This includes the way history is written, the way a group is spoken about, the vocabulary allocated to a group, and the questions asked in research on that group. This is then used to justify future actions against that group.

Research based on a selected demographic characteristic, such as sexuality or gender identity, should be considered carefully, as it holds the potential to contribute to this othering process. As consumers and creators of research, clinical neuropsychologists may (perhaps inadvertently) become the agent of othering. This contributes to the minoritisation of certain groups, where their mistreatment, marginalisation, and erasure becomes justified by 'the data'. Furthermore, the allocation of the quality of difference is located in the minoritised group. The implication being that it is the burden of that group to endure the inconveniences of an inflexible majority that prioritises its own needs and perspectives in the asking of research questions and the allocation of resources.

The Evidence Base

There have been decades of research in psychology and neuroscience on cisgender/sex differences in cognitive function and brain structure. These have been highly publicised and have been taken as established fact by the scientific community and the public at large (Rippon, 2020). The assumption that male and female brains are different (called 'sexual dimorphism') in structure and function between cis men and women gives rise to the expectation that differences should be found for individuals who defy gendered norms.

Several papers have recently discredited the dimorphism of the amygdala and hippocampus (Tan et al., 2016; Marwha et al., 2017). In addition, a recent comprehensive review by Eliot et al. (2021) considered in detail the literature and found that there is almost no evidence of functional or structural sexual dimorphism. They found that publication bias, highly flawed method, and lack of replicability (amongst others) have misrepresented the data. Eliot et al. (2021) found consistent support for only one or two clinically/functionally insignificant, possibly dimorphic findings, e.g., larger average male brain size or the presence and size of the interthalamic adhesion (which is absent in 2–22% of healthy brains). They also provide evidence that where cognitive differences do occur (e.g., rotation, verbal fluency) in the literature, these do not have a neural basis.

Another confounding factor in this type of research is plasticity and the brain's tendency to adapt to how it is used. A demonstration of this principle can be found in the London taxi driver study by Woollett et al. (2009). A brain that shows any gender-based differences in structure and function may be a brain that has been so structured due to how it has been functioning according to the requirement of the developmental environment, which is determined in large part by the gender identity assigned at birth. In support of the significance of this effect, Eliot et al. (2021) discuss that the differences in cognitive functioning found between cis men and cis women do not appear to be demonstrable in youth, i.e., they are not innate. Where these differences do emerge, there is significant overlap at the group comparison level between male and female performance (Rippon, 2020), and one does not have to have a genetically or structurally 'male' brain or body in order to show male profiles of performance. More broadly in terms of scope and more specifically to the SOGIRD communities, Hyde et al. (2019) provide five challenges to the assumption of the gender binary, summarising research from neuroscience, behavioural neuroendocrinology, cisgender-based psychological research, transgender psychological research, and developmental psychology.

In summary, there is cause to be highly sceptical of gender-based brain research. Thus, the challenges posed to neuropsychologists working with SOGIRD clients, for example, which gender norms to use in assessment, cannot be easily solved by adherence to research that supports gender-essentialist ideals when the entire basis for gender as a fundamental way to understand our neurocognitive nature is questionable.

Assessment and Formulation

The assessment approaches familiar to the clinical neuropsychologist should not be considered inappropriate to use with SOGIRD clients. Fundamentally, there should be few issues with testing or falsifying hypotheses about brain function and the diagnosis of neurocognitive, neuroaffective, or neurobehavioural syndromes with standardised assessments. As mentioned, the expectation of group differences based on the assumption of dimorphic sex in cognition and brain structure are being convincingly and increasingly discredited. Thus, the basis for which one should expect differences based on sexuality and gender identity has been significantly undermined. Furthermore, many of the core assessment tests and batteries (the TOPF 2, WAIS, WMS, Brixton Hayling, BADS, RBANS, DKEFS, BDI, BAI, HADS, ACE-R) do not, in fact, use gendered norms.

As with any medical treatment, the assessing clinician needs to explore the effects of any medical procedures or medications and ascertain whether it is appropriate to assess the client if they are undergoing any kind of incomplete treatment. For trans individuals, this often means a discussion about surgeries and hormone therapy. However, the evidence on whether hormone medications specifically affect cognition is currently unclear (Keo-Meier & Fitzgerald, 2017; Trittschuh et al., 2018). For gay men enquiring about serostatus (HIV) can be important (Bloch et al., 2016), especially for those who are older and who may not have had access to antiviral medications for some time.

Whilst the rationale for neurocognitive assessment may be less affected by issues of gender identity and sexuality, it is known that SOGIRD clients can score higher on personality inventories according to which gender norms are used, and one must consider the established impact of increased incidence of mood and mental health difficulty on cognition (Borgogna et al., 2019). These additional concerns require knowledge of the SOGIRD individual's background to direct assessment questions in interview to ascertain the extent to which a finding of cognitive, behavioural, or affective dysfunction may be affected by or attributed to non-neurocognitive factors.

To compliment mainstream assessment approaches, the clinical neuropsychologist can consider the minority stress hypothesis (Meyer, 1995), which outlines the role of oppression-based stress factors on mental health, and the gender minority stress and resilience measure (Testa et al., 2015). Together these adjuncts to clinical practice can be used to assess and formulate in a SOGIRD-sensitive manner. Keo-Meier and Fitzgerald (2017) also suggest embedding practice within a gender affirmative model (GAM), which takes as an assumption that gender nonconformity is not the cause, result, or symptom of a pathological process.

As outlined in the American Psychological Association guidance (2020), the evidence is scant for SOGIRD communities, and one must be wary of attempting to use norms and procedures that are not fully evidenced. This is especially so in contexts where a SOGIRD individual may be misrepresented to the lay consumer, e.g., jurors and judges in legal contexts, as having been 'thoroughly assessed', when in fact the tools used are more likely to be invalid for this population. It does not serve the SOGIRD communities to use a 'do-what-we-can-and-accept-the-error' approach, which would not be acceptable practice for cis-het individuals. It is incumbent upon the clinical neuropsychologist to uphold parity of standards between cis-het and SOGIRD clients and to refuse to offer substandard, othering, minoritising practice.

Treatment and Rehabilitation

The interventions of a clinical neuropsychologist can vary widely, from rehabilitation and psychoeducation to psychotherapy and family sessions. A full discussion of each of these areas of practice is not possible, both because of a lack of research for SOGIRD individuals and an abundance of different interventive and therapeutic approaches to consider at the conceptual level. However, useful guidance can be found in the adjacent psychotherapeutic literature, which can facilitate intervention with SOGIRD clients. It is of more use to consider the position from which we interact and intervene, rather than differentiating treatment approaches based on socially constructed concepts of gender identity and sexual orientation, which may or may not apply to the client.

Davies (2000) describes an approach to working with lesbian, gay, and bisexual clients, which he refers to as affirmative therapy. He outlines the core concepts as:

- '[R]espect for the client's sexual orientation,
- [Respect] for personal integrity,
- [Respect] for lifestyle and culture, together with
- Respectful attitudes and beliefs.'

(Davies, 2000, p. 56)

Additional subsequent considerations for the clinician working with SOGIRD clients are:

- The therapist should have an awareness and be at ease with their own sexuality,
- The therapist should be aware of the context of oppression experienced by SOGIRD individuals, and
- The therapist should be aware of the socio-political history of SOGIRD peoples and the diversity across these groups.

At first glance, it may be hard to relate this guidance to the assessment and treatment of neurocognitive dysfunction. However, consider that the clinical neuropsychologist draws on information from a great number of different areas (e.g., personality, mental health, behaviour, family/ systems, education, attachment, occupation, medicine, neuroimaging, standardised scores, etc.). The meaning we might make in integrating these different types of data is vulnerable to the assumptions, biases, and limitations of understanding that we hold as individuals. For example, a clinician unaware that lesbians are at increased risk of sexual violence might misattribute a reluctance to leave the house as social anxiety. A lack of awareness of the acceptance of open relationships amongst gay men as a valid format for relationships might be interpreted as post-traumatic hypersexuality where it coincides with relationship problems as a result of a brain injury.

It is also important to consider how intervention may be experienced by clients and what their previous experience of clinicians might be. One in twenty SOGIRD individuals have experienced some kind of 'conversion therapy', and 19% of these unethical interventions were provided by healthcare or medical professionals, making them the second largest provider after religious groups (Government Equalities Office, 2019). Survivors of these approaches may thus be suspicious of clinicians whose job is to measure and make judgement of function as compared against preconceived ideas of normality.

Davies and Neal (1996) explore a number of different models of psychotherapy in the context of working with SOGIRD individuals. De Cecco's (2020) foreword in Jon Gonsiorek's *Guide to Psychotherapy with Gay and Lesbian Clients* raises the importance of work with SOGIRD groups not becoming pathologised. In the context of recent developments in the understanding of sex research on brain structure and function not indicating dimorphism, this makes sense. There is no need for a separate science of psychotherapy or rehabilitation with SOGIRD individuals, but there is a need to situate the political act of intervention in the context from which our clients are operating. For example, therapeutic endeavours which make sense to cis-het individuals, such as 'radical acceptance' (dialectical behaviour therapy) and 'thought challenging' (cognitive behaviour therapy) must be used carefully with SOGIRD individuals where the world around them is consistently oppressive, non-changing, and harmful.

How much can a person radically accept before they learn helplessness? How many thoughts can one reasonably challenge without generating internal conflict and self-directed anger? Where does social change come from if we have erased the anger? The ubiquitous psychotherapeutic construction of anger and rage as 'understandable, nothing to be ashamed of, but nonetheless something to move away from' at the social level can be a patronising diminution of the obstacles that minoritized groups must overcome on a daily basis. Assessment, diagnosis, and therapy can quickly become forms of social control and political disarmament enacted by clinicians and educators on behalf of an oppressive and often dangerous society. As clinicians we must be careful of isolating the individual from their context without also enabling the context to be addressed.

Towards Cultural Competence

'Cultural competence' is a term adopted from social work and health-care practice that originally referred to the ability to work sensitively and effectively across cultures and ethnic groups (Sue, 1998). In recent years the field has advanced beyond the adoption of a flexible epistemology and detailed awareness of the characteristics of minoritised groups, to using scientific method, to identifying specific risk and resilience factors in treatment outcomes for different communities – the modifications that these lead to being referred to as 'cultural adaptations' (DeAngelis, 2015).

Cultural competence is increasingly being used to understand SOGIRD service provision issues in the US but less so, at present, in the UK. And whilst there has been some progress, questions remain. Why do we require a separate field of culturally specific study for specific groups? Surely the question is why are the models used not universally applicable? At what stage does bias occur in our models and services?

For clinical neuropsychology, these are more than questions of equality and diversity. As a science, neuropsychology should place great emphasis on identifying systematic errors and biases in our study and practice that favour one group of people, especially when that knowledge is digested by the public as a universal, scientific fact.

Where the issue is less attributable to flaws in models and more about the clinical application of a model to a minoritised SOGIRD group, some tools have been created for clinicians, such as the LGBT Ally Identity Measure (Jones et al., 2014) and the LGBT Development of Clinical Skills Scale (Bidell, 2017). Furthermore, to situate one's intervention in a formulation that is inclusive, sensitive, and affirmative, the clinical neuropsychologist can look to the social constructionist therapies (e.g., social constructionist systemic therapy, narrative therapy) and frameworks, such as the Coordinated Management of Meaning (Cronen et al., 1979) and the Approach-Method-Technique model (Burnham, 1999).

Conclusion

At present it appears that what clinical neuropsychology as a discipline has to offer SOGIRD individuals may be limited by the evidence base and the socio-political context within which that research has taken place. More work needs to be undertaken to expand our knowledge, and the SOGIRD communities should lead the direction of this research. As a profession there must be care taken over repeating the historical mistakes of the field of psychology, which, when politicised, has caused enduring harm.

However, what clinical neuropsychologists have to offer as individuals is considerable. We improve our practices for all individuals by adopting the 'null' position and saying where we cannot offer an opinion, being accurate about the limitations we must work within, and insisting that we adhere to the same standards expected by the cis-het community.

References

American Psychological Association. (2020, December). Psychological and Neuropsychological Assessment with Transgender and Gender Nonbinary Adults. *American Psychological Association.* https://www.apa.org/pi/lgbt/resources/transgender-gender-nonbinary.

Bell vs Tavistock and Portman NHS Foundation Trust. (2020). [2020] EWHC 3274 (Admin). Retrieved from https://www.bailii.org/ew/cases/EWHC/Admin/2020/3274.html.

Bell vs Tavistock and Portman NHS Foundation Trust. (2021). [2021] EWCA Civ 1363. Retrieved from https://www.bailii.org/ew/cases/EWCA/Civ/2021/1363.html.

Bidell, M. P. (2017). The Lesbian, Gay, Bisexual, and Transgender Development of Clinical Skills Scale (LGBT-DOCSS): Establishing a New Interdisciplinary Self-Assessment for Health Providers. *Journal of Homosexuality, 64*(10), 1432–1460. DOI: 10.1080/00918369.2017.1321389.

Bloch, M., Kamminga, J., Jayewardene, A., Bailey, M., Carberry, A., Vincent, T., Quan, D., Maruff, P., Brew, B., & Cysique, L. A. (2016). A Screening Strategy for HIV-Associated Neurocognitive Disorders That Accurately Identifies Patients Requiring Neurological Review. *Clinical Infectious Diseases, 63*(5), 687–693. DOI: 10.1093/cid/ciw399.

Borgogna, N. C., McDermott, R. C., Aita, S. L., & Kridel, M. M. (2019). Anxiety and depression across gender and sexual minorities: Implications for transgender, gender nonconforming, pansexual, demisexual, asexual, queer, and questioning individuals. *Psychology of Sexual Orientation and Gender Diversity, 6*(1), 54–63. DOI: 10.1037/sgd0000306.

Burnham, J. (1999). Approach, Method, Technique: Making distinctions and creating connections. *Human Systems: The Journal of Systemic Consultation and Management, 3*(1), 3–26.

Butler, C., O'Donovan, A., & Shaw, E. (2010). *Sex, Sexuality and Therapeutic Practice: A Manual for Therapists and Trainers* (1st ed.). Routledge.

Butler, J. (1990). *Gender Trouble: Feminism and the Subversion of Identity* (Routledge Classics) (1st ed.). Routledge.

Cronen, V. E., Pearce, W. B., & Harris, L. M. (1979). The logic of the coordinated management of meaning: A rules-based approach to the first course in interpersonal communication. *Communication Education, 28*(1), 22–38. DOI: 10.1080/03634527909378327.

Davies, D. (2000). *Therapeutic Perspectives On Working With Lesbian, Gay and Bisexual Clients* (Pink Therapy) (1st ed.). Open University Press.

Davies, D., & Neal, C. (1996). *Pink Therapy* (1st ed.). Open University Press.

De Beauvoir, S. (2021). *The Second Sex*. Tingle Books. (Original work published in 1949 as *Le Deuxième Sexe*)

DeAngelis, T. (2015). In search of cultural competence. *American Psychological Association: Monitor on Psychology, 64*(3), 64.

De Cecco, J. P. (2000). Foreward. In J. Gonsiorek (Ed.), *Guide to Psychotherapy with Gay and Lesbian Clients* (pp. 1–2). Routledge.

Drydakis, N. (2021). Sexual Orientation and Earnings: A Meta-Analysis 2012–2020. *SSRN Electronic Journal*. DOI: 10.2139/ssrn.3874368.

Eliot, L., Ahmed, A., Khan, H., & Patel, J. (2021). Dump the "dimorphism": Comprehensive synthesis of human brain studies reveals few male-female differences beyond size. *Neuroscience & Biobehavioral Reviews, 125*, 667–697. DOI: 10.1016/j.neubiorev.2021.02.026.

Fischer, M. (2021). Making Black Trans Lives Matter. *QED: A Journal in GLBTQ Worldmaking, 8*(1), 111. DOI: 10.14321/qed.8.1.0111.

Florida State Senate. (2022, January). *Parental Rights in Education*. https://www.flsenate.gov/Session/Bill/2022/1557/?Tab=BillHistory.

Gelman, S. A. (2005). *The Essential Child: Origins of Essentialism in Everyday Thought* (Oxford Series in Cognitive Development). Oxford University Press.

Government Equalities Office. (2019). *National LGBT Survey*. https://www.gov.uk/government/publications/national-lgbt-survey-summary-report.

Grayling, A. C. (2021). *The History of Philosophy* (Reprint ed.). Penguin Books.

Human Dignity Trust. (2022). *Map of Countries that Criminalise LGBT People*. Retrieved 9 April 2022 from https://www.humandignitytrust.org/lgbt-the-law/map-of-criminalisation.

Human Rights Campaign. (2021). *Fatal Violence Against the Transgender and Gender Non-Conforming Community in 2021*. https://www.hrc.org/resources/fatal-violence-against-the-transgender-and-gender-non-conforming-community-in-2021.

Human Rights Watch. (2018, December). *No Support: Russia's 'Gay Propaganda' Law Imperils LGBT Youth*. https://www.hrw.org/report/2018/12/12/no-support/russias-gay-propaganda-law-imperils-lgbt-youth.

Hunte, B. (2021, October 11). 'Don't Punish Me For Who I Am': Huge Jump in Anti-LGBTQ Hate Crime Reports in UK. *Vice*. Retrieved 9 March 2022 from https://www.vice.com/en/article/4avkyw/anti-lgbtq-hate-crime-reports-increase-in-six-years.

Hyde, J. S., Bigler, R. S., Joel, D., Tate, C. C., & van Anders, S. M. (2019). The future of sex and gender in psychology: Five challenges to the gender binary. *American Psychologist, 74*(2), 171–193. DOI: 10.1037/amp0000307.

Izzard, S. (2000). Psychoanalytic Psychotherapy. In D. Davies & C. Neal (Eds.), *Therapeutic Perspectives On Working With Lesbian, Gay and Bisexual Clients* (Pink Therapy) (1st ed.) (pp. 106–121). Open University Press.

Jones, K. N., Brewster, M. E., & Jones, J. A. (2014). The creation and validation of the LGBT Ally Identity Measure. *Psychology of Sexual Orientation and Gender Diversity, 1*(2), 181–195. DOI: 10.1037/sgd0000033.

Jowett, A., Brady, G., Goodman, S., Pillinger, C., & Bradley, L. (2021). *Conversion Therapy: An evidence assessment and qualitative study.* The Government Equalities Office. https://www.gov.uk/government/publications/conversion-therapy-an-evidence-assessment-and-qualitative-study/conversion-therapy-an-evidence-assessment-and-qualitative-study.

Keo-Meier, C. L., & Fitzgerald, K. M. (2017). Affirmative Psychological Testing and Neurocognitive Assessment with Transgender Adults. *Psychiatric Clinics of North America, 40*(1), 51–64. DOI: 10.1016/j.psc.2016.10.011.

LGBT Foundation. (2020, February). *Hidden Figures: LGBT Health Inequalities in the UK.* https://lgbt.foundation/hiddenfigures.

Mandalaywala, T. M., Amodio, D. M., & Rhodes, M. (2017). Essentialism Promotes Racial Prejudice by Increasing Endorsement of Social Hierarchies. *Social Psychological and Personality Science, 9*(4), 461–469. DOI: 10.1177/1948550617707020.

Margaret Thatcher's Anti-Gay Speech (1:00 min). (2013, April 12). *YouTube.* Retrieved 26 March 2022 from https://www.youtube.com/watch?v=8VRRWuryb4k.

Marwha, D., Halari, M., & Eliot, L. (2017). Meta-analysis reveals a lack of sexual dimorphism in human amygdala volume. *NeuroImage, 147,* 282–294. DOI: 10.1016/j.neuroimage.2016.12.021.

Maurice, E. P. (2019, November 5). Piers Morgan will not face Ofcom investigation after nearly 1,000 viewers complained about him identifying 'as a penguin'. *PinkNews.* https://www.pinknews.co.uk/2019/11/05/piers-morgan-good-morning-britain-ofcom-two-spirit-penguin.

McLean, C. (2021). The Growth of the Anti-Transgender Movement in the United Kingdom: The Silent Radicalization of the British Electorate. *International Journal of Sociology, 51*(6), 473–482. DOI: 10.1080/00207659.2021.1939946.

Meyer, I. H. (1995). Minority Stress and Mental Health in Gay Men. *Journal of Health and Social Behavior, 36*(1), 38–56. DOI: 10.2307/2137286.

Office of National Statistics. (2020, October). *Ethnicity Pay Gaps: 2019.* https://www.ons.gov.uk/employmentandlabourmarket/peopleinwork/earningsandworkinghours/articles/ethnicitypaygapsingreatbritain/2019.

Petter, O. (2020, June 15). JK Rowling criticised over 'transphobic' tweet about menstruation. *The Independent.* https://www.independent.co.uk/life-style/jk-rowling-tweet-women-menstruate-people-transphobia-twitter-a9552866.html.

Rippon, G. (2020). *The Gendered Brain: The new neuroscience that shatters the myth of the female brain.* Vintage.

Smith, G. (2004). Treatments of homosexuality in Britain since the 1950s – An oral history: The experience of patients. *BMJ, 328*(7437), 427. DOI: 10.1136/bmj.37984.442419.ee.

Spivak, G. C. (1985). The Rani of Sirmur: An Essay in Reading the Archives. *History and Theory, 24*(3), 247–272. DOI: 10.2307/2505169.

Stonewall. (2017, September). *LGBT Britain Hate Crime and Discrimination.* https://www.stonewall.org.uk/lgbt-britain-hate-crime-and-discrimination.

Sue, S. (1998). In search of cultural competence in psychotherapy and counseling. *American Psychologist, 53*(4), 440–448. DOI: 10.1037/0003–066x.53.4.440.

Tan, A., Ma, W., Vira, A., Marwha, D., & Eliot, L. (2016). The human hippocampus is not sexually-dimorphic: Meta-analysis of structural MRI volumes. *NeuroImage, 124,* 350–366. DOI: 10.1016/j.neuroimage.2015.08.050.

Testa, R. J., Habarth, J., Peta, J., Balsam, K., & Bockting, W. (2015). Development of the Gender Minority Stress and Resilience Measure. *Psychology of Sexual Orientation and Gender Diversity, 2*(1), 65–77. DOI: 10.1037/sgd0000081.

Trittschuh, E. H., Parmenter, B. A., Clausell, E. R., Mariano, M. J., & Reger, M. A. (2018). Conducting neuropsychological assessment with transgender individuals. *The Clinical Neuropsychologist, 32*(8), 1393–1410. DOI: 10.1080/13854046.2018.144063.

UK Government. (1988). *Local Government Act.* https://www.legislation.gov.uk/ukpga/1988/9/contents.

Woollett, K., Spiers, H. J., & Maguire, E. A. (2009). Talent in the taxi: A model system for exploring expertise. *Philosophical Transactions of the Royal Society B: Biological Sciences, 364*(1522), 1407–1416. DOI: 10.1098/rstb.2008.0288.

Yakushko, O. (2019). Eugenics and its evolution in the history of western psychology: A critical archival review. *Psychotherapy and Politics International, 17*(2), e1495. DOI: 10.1002/ppi.1495.

Part 4

Socio-Political Sensitivity in Leadership

11 Leading with Humility

Lorraine Haye, Eva Sundin and Masuma Rahim

Introduction

For some psychologists, being framed as a 'leader' can feel self-aggrandising. We enter the NHS as newly qualified clinicians at a relatively high pay grade, but often with considerably less experience than our nursing and therapy colleagues. Even the most confident clinical psychologist will soon realise that they exist within a complex system – a system inhabited by patients, family members, social workers, commissioners, therapists, rehab nurses, physicians, neuronavigators, domiciliary care staff, and Best Interests assessors. How, then, can one take on the mantle of a 'leader'? More importantly, how can one keep in check the tendency to want to lead or to be in power when we know that healthcare professionals should be more concerned with democratising power?

The distinction between 'Big L' Leadership and 'Little L' leadership can be useful to appease some of these internal conflicts. 'Big L' Leadership represents formally recognised leadership roles held by people who are expected to lead because that is the explicit requirement of their role, e.g., consultant psychologist, clinical lead, etc. 'Little L' leadership represents leading by example through influence and stepping up when things need to be done, regardless of job designation. The role of a clinical psychologist is fundamentally about using influence to shape change at the level of the individual, team, organisation, and beyond (British Psychological Society, 2007). Therefore, leadership is an inescapable part of the professional identity.

Clinical neuropsychologists can use professional influence to bolster good practice in healthcare organisations through bringing about psychologically informed care as a complement to (or disruption of) dominant medical models. Furthermore, psychological expertise can hold people accountable, build alliances, and encourage professional growth. The high demand for increased efficiency, productivity, and improved quality of care requires that clinical leadership extends beyond day-to-day healthcare provision. In the current socio-political climate, it is more essential than ever that psychologists work with an appreciation of difference, diversity, inclusion, and equity. Historically,

DOI: 10.4324/9781003309819-15

the concept of cultural competency emphasised that a level of knowledge and understanding of diversity was crucial when working with people from diverse backgrounds. While 'cultural competency' implies a set standard to be attained, Tervalon and Murray-García's (1998) concept of cultural humility outlines an ongoing dynamic process. This concept focuses on the self rather than the 'other' and emphasises the need for personal reflection, growth, and learning collaboratively from team members, patients, and their families. Additional key features of cultural humility include a willingness to suspend what one thinks one knows, introspection, lifelong learning, actively addressing power imbalances and inequity by developing and nurturing mutually beneficial partnerships, and institutional accountability. Tervalon and Murray-García (1998) stressed that 'cultural' does not refer solely to racial and ethnic identity. Consequently, within the research literature, the 'cultural' part of cultural humility is used in reference to various underserved communities.

In recent years, humility has been explored as a quality more generally in healthcare. It can broadly be understood by the following quote:

> Humility is not self-deprecation ... Humility represents wisdom ... Humility is knowing you are smart, but not all-knowing. It is accepting that you have personal power, but are not omnipotent ... Inherent in humility resides an open and receptive mind ... it leaves us more open to learn from others and refrains from seeing issues and people only in blacks and whites.
>
> (Templeton, 1997, pp. 162–163)

Evidence has shown that humility is important within healthcare settings for successful inter-professional collaboration. It can create healthier and more effective organisational cultures, develop employees' potential and boost team morale, job satisfaction, and performance (Yang et al., 2019). Clinician humility positively predicted patient satisfaction, trust, self-reported health, and therapy outcomes (Huynh & Dicke-Bohemann, 2020; Owen et al., 2016). An explanation of these beneficial outcomes is that humility enhances team innovation by fostering the shared perception among team members that they are able to speak up.

Within the context of neuropsychology, the idea of embracing humility as a central way of working might be aversive for some. It may seem antithetical to the journey of becoming a clinical neuropsychologist, which entails extensive training and assessment to demonstrate knowledge, skill, and expertise. In this chapter, we will describe how leading with humility can provide a valuable foundation for an approach to working with people with acquired brain injuries.

Leading with Humility   171

Applications of Humility in Neuropsychology

Assessment

The psychological professions have committed grave and well-documented crimes in the name of science, not least our involvement in the eugenics movement, which aimed to 'improve the natural, physical, mental, and temperamental qualities of the human family' (Norrgard, 2008, p. 170). Its role in creating and maintaining racial disparities is much more recent than many may like to think: in the 1960s and 70s, British educational and clinical psychologists were part of a programme supported by the Inner London Education Authority to remove Black children from mainstream schools and enrol them in 'special' schools for the 'educationally subnormal'. It was a policy that was systematically racist and oppressive, and one that was defeated only because of the efforts of grassroots campaigners such as Gus John; Bernard Coard; and Mollie Hunte, a Black educational psychologist; and the Black community (Coard, 1971).

It is not difficult to see how this came about when one considers the history of the profession. The early days of clinical psychology training required the fledgling profession to claim an identity and mark its territory in the health sciences. Hans Eysenck, one of the key figures in the development of clinical psychology as a profession in the UK, stated in 1971 that:

> this discovery of a strong genetic involvement in the determination of individual differences in IQ between members of a given population is an essential precondition for going on to argue in favour of the genetic determination (in part at least) of racial differences in IQ ... I am not a racist for believing it possible that Negroes may have special innate gifts for certain athletic events, such as sprints, or for certain musical forms of expression ... Nor am I a racist for seriously considering the possibility that the demonstrated inferiority of American Negroes on tests of intelligence may, in part, be due to genetic causes.
>
> (Eysenck, 1971, p. 112, p. 6)

Fifty years later, much of Eysenck's work has been discredited, and we know that genetically determined differences in race and IQ are 'a priori unlikely rather than likely' (Colman, 2016, p. 186). We also know that structural inequalities, including poverty, overcrowding, and limited access to educational opportunities, significantly predict scores on psychometric tests (Barnett, 1998). We have learned that our assessment tools simply do not demonstrate reliability and validity for many of the people we see (Casaletto & Heaton, 2017). Developmental delay, communication impairments, education, and medication side effects all affect the extent to which patients are able to engage in assessment. Additionally, for people unused to being asked to sit at a table and undertake several hours' worth of pencil-and-paper tasks (or those traumatised by their experiences of it), the assessment process is likely to be extremely challenging (Nell, 1999).

Of course, neuropsychological assessment is not limited to psychometrics. Good neuropsychology is systemic in its approach and should cast the net wide for information that can contribute to the formulation. Brain injuries cause huge amounts of upheaval and distress. The impact on role, identity, financial stability, and relationships has been well-documented, as has the data regarding the prevalence of depression and anxiety post-brain injury (Sariaslan et al., 2016). Subsequently, if neuropsychology is fundamentally a human and humane science, we must handle patients gently, particularly during the assessment process.

Power should never be far from the mind of the healthcare professional. Irrespective of our personal demographics, we often have significant power within clinical relationships. We have knowledge, skills, and sometimes expertise which our patients do not have. We use language which reflects our specialism but which also serves to cloak our thinking and practice in mystery. We can give diagnoses and prognoses which are life-altering. It is vital, therefore, that we wield that power carefully, thoughtfully, and in a way which the patient and the wider system can bear.

David Smail (2005) describes 'the impress of power', distinguishing the person from the proximal influences, including education, employment, relationships, and housing, and distal influences, such as politics, economics, and culture, that affect their day-to-day lives. He describes the social environment as being the milieu which most substantially affects patients' lives, and reminds us that, whilst we as professionals may have some impact or influence, this will pale in comparison to the impact of social and material factors.

In practical terms, this means that our assessments have to be sensitive to patients' social, cultural, and historical contexts. It also means that clinicians have to acknowledge how little we know about patients when we first meet them. Whether a patient has been referred for therapy for mood-related difficulties, behavioural management, or neuropsychological assessment, there is likely to be a system of family members and carers who have an in-depth understanding of the patient and their needs. They may even have their own working formulation to explain the patient's difficulties. Engaging with the entirety of that system to identify and work with the information held within it is vital.

There are clear limits to the impact our assessments (and the resultant findings) can make. In our experience, patients and family members often come to assessment appointments reporting specific cognitive and functional changes. Neuropsychological assessment simply serves to confirm those changes. In essence, although our assessment may provide useful recommendations or be a necessary part of their journey through the neurosciences pathway, it may not add much of interest to the patient's own understanding of their difficulties.

Neuropsychology is often described as detective work, but we prefer to think of it as the skilled application of practical problem-solving. Ultimately, the job of the neuropsychologist is to gather the information required to be able to clearly identify the problem. Only then can anything approximating useful intervention be offered. Since people are complex, their problems are frequently complex. The net must be cast wide if patients and their families are to get effective care and treatment. After all, 'a good decision is based on knowledge and not on numbers' (Plato, 1871).

Formulation

Clinical neuropsychologists work with people who represent a wide range of patient presentations and health conditions. Across this work, the clinical assessment, cognitive testing, and diagnosis are common strands to identify cognitive, emotional, and behavioural consequences of neurological conditions. These procedures produce a large amount of information which is at least partly inconsistent. It is here that the formulation plays a crucial role as it pulls together the disconnected pieces of information to a coherent narrative. Some clinical scholars even propose that it represents a skill that sets psychologists apart from other health professionals (Macniven, 2018). But, what is a formulation, and how do psychologists weigh, sort, and summarise all the information gained from the history taking, clinical assessment, and cognitive testing? A classic definition was presented by Tracy Eells (1997) decades ago: A formulation is a

> hypothesis about the causes, precipitants, and maintaining influences of a person's psychological, interpersonal, and behavioural problems ... it serves as a blueprint guiding treatment, as a marker for change, [and] as a structure for enabling the therapist to understand the patient better.
>
> (p. 2)

If we unpack Eells's definition, we can overview its key elements. First, a formulation is a hypothesis. At times it is made up of initial suppositions and guesswork, at other times it is something akin to a belief. It is a way of summarising and synthesising various bits of information that are seemingly incoherent and creating a narrative that is clear to understand for the patient and other health professionals. The formulation can provide a road map for treatment, and it can be checked against treatment-interfering behaviour and patient change that can be hypothesised given the formulation. Critically important is that the formulation provides the psychologist and the clinical team with an enhanced understanding of the patient, which in turn enables the growth of empathy.

The patient's role in the development of the formulation is variable. At one end, the patient is assigned the traditional patient role as a passive recipient of care (Wagner et al., 2005). At the other end, the patient is invited to contribute their perceptions of what is causing, precipitating, and persevering the health problems as well as what interventions might be beneficial for them.

The role of the patient is largely determined by the psychologist's leadership style. When the psychologist views and communicates the formulation as her or his fixed belief, little room is offered to the patient or the team to engage in joint discussions. Such top-down communication of the formulation can manifest itself in the power dynamics between the psychologist and their patient as well as between the psychologist and other team members. In this context, the patient is assigned a passive role in the interaction with the psychologist, which may show itself in a laid-back attitude in treatment and limited engagement in health-promoting behaviour. Such processes are documented in the literature across a wide variety of psychological interventions (see Del Re et al., 2012 for a meta-analysis).

When the psychologist is mindful that the formulation is just one of many possible explanations of the patient's problems, this awareness can help the psychologist to avoid the trap of wrongly assuming they have obtained the truth of a matter. The humble psychologist can then share with the patient that they only have access to partial information about the patient and that they take risks when they arrive at decisions. Therefore, for the humble psychologist, the patient's active engagement in the development of the formulation is not only welcome, but also of vital importance for establishing the accuracy of the formulation, which can guide the treatment.

The humility with which the unpretentious psychologist works on the formulation as a joint task with the patient can enhance a collaborative relationship with the patient (Spencer et al., 2019). In turn, although the psychologist's role in the treatment relationship is more important for psychologist and patient experience of the relationship (Del Re et al., 2012), the quality rather than the quantity of the patient's input is also important (Schmidt & Woolaway-Bickel, 2000).

Intervention

Interventions aimed directly at individuals within a neuropsychology context can refer to neuropsychological rehabilitation which involves supporting with compensatory strategies. There is also psychological therapy and psychoeducation often aimed at addressing mood, behavioural changes, and general adjustment. When setting clear goals for intervention it is important to aim for collaboration and understand the power dynamics inherent in the work. For instance, when someone is in the early stages of adjusting to an acquired brain injury and might be eager for any and all help, it can be easy to set generic goals that are not personally meaningful to the person.

Good psychoeducation is imperative to help patients understand not only the multitude of ways in which an acquired brain injury can impact their life but also the scope for what can be covered as part of an intervention. For example, sexual dysfunction after a stroke is common but frequently unaddressed by healthcare providers, with counselling indicated as the primary intervention of choice (Stein et al., 2013; Calabrò & Bramanti, 2014). Many of the causes of sexual dysfunction relate to psychosocial factors and are rarely due to the result of brain damage. Yet professionals' perceptions that they do not have adequate skills in addressing sexuality, their personal level of (dis)comfort with the topic, and unhelpful attitudes towards stroke survivors and sexuality create a series of barriers to limit opportunities for engagement (Richards et al., 2016). Sexuality is an important aspect of quality of life and should be considered as part of holistic care. This has been recognised in the national clinical guideline for stroke, which recommends further research into sexuality in the context of rehabilitation (Rudd et al., 2017).

Our own anxieties about discussing or dealing with certain topics as part of rehabilitation treatment may mean we avoid having important conversations. This may be because we worry about what intervention we could possibly offer, so we do not begin to explore what the intervention could look like, when in reality it may be similar to or likely fit with existing models of how we work. For instance, the PLISSIT model (Annon, 1976) is a stepped-care approach to working with sexual problems that is not too dissimilar to the stepped-care model used to identify the appropriate level of psychological intervention required in mental health. PLISSIT stands for: Permission (P) Limited Information (LI), Specific Suggestions (SS), and Intensive Therapy (IT). The first step of 'Permission' refers to creating opportunities for discussion of the issue. This alone can often be enough to address the problem, with further intervention being unnecessary. However, similar to the stepped-care model where professionals can often bypass lower-level interventions to deploy more intensive ones, many people may miss the Permission stage and proceed with information-giving or signposting elsewhere. A willingness to continuously seek information, develop our knowledge, and pursue personal development to broaden our personal comfort in relation to the things we are less confident about is important in being able to improve the flexibility with which we can provide support.

The idea that any intervention offered is better than nothing can be harmful at worst and arrogant at best. It is important to hold that not every person will benefit from direct neuropsychology or clinical psychology intervention. Additionally, the timing of when we offer an intervention can differentiate between it being something helpful or harmful. In a desire to raise the profile of psychology, services can be expanded to provide interventions beyond the skills and resources available in the service. Strategic thinking should not compromise patient care. This can increase burnout, frustration, and moral injury for clinicians, as it falls on them to deliver the undeliverable.

Regardless of the type of intervention or therapeutic modality used, it is imperative to understand and be able to work with issues of transference and countertransference. This is important to avoid replicating and aggravating attachment traumas. Regardless of whether patients have premorbid mental health difficulties, the experience of navigating various pathways in healthcare and engagement with a range of professionals can be really traumatising. At the absolute minimum we should give due consideration to the patient experience from referral to discharge in our service area and the pacing of multi-disciplinary team (MDT) engagement.

Groups are another means through which we can offer interventions. They can be an efficient way to stretch resources, they can help people connect to others with shared experiences, and they can create an opportunity for people to re-engage with their community at a time when they may feel isolated and disconnected. Informed consent is very important, with problems arising if a group is offered as the only option for intervention. There would need to be careful consideration on whether the group composition is based on diagnosis, demographic characteristics, or specific issues, such as fatigue, memory, etc. If it is the latter, it is important to then make space for consideration of the nuances of people's experiences, such as the intersections between adjusting to life with an unseen disability alongside class, sexuality, race, gender, etc. This also needs to be reflected in the breadth and range of materials and the examples that we use in groups. The running of groups is a whole skill set in itself and can often be a responsibility designated to trainees and assistant psychologists. Therefore, it is important that we support pre-qualified psychologists to understand and address some of the group dynamics that will emerge. This can help to preserve the relational benefits of a group intervention and avoid the group being reduced solely to an information-giving platform.

Working with Systems/Consultation

MDTs, Families, and Other Organisations

Brain injuries do not happen to people; they happen to families. The sequalae of neurological conditions and brain injury on partners, children, and parents are well documented (Whiffin et al., 2021). Our experience is that even the best neuropsychological treatment is ineffective if

knowledge and responsibility is not shared with the system and if rehabilitation is not made the responsibility of everyone within that system,
rather than being held by a small group of experienced professionals.

There are evident challenges to working in partnership with family
members in the acute phase. Initially, there is the patient's experience in
addition to the highly distressing medical interventions, such as surgeries
and scans. There are also complex legal issues, such as mental capacity,
alongside behaviour and personality changes, sometimes subtle and often marked. To come to terms with the fact that your partner or parent
is not the person they were before the injury is difficult for many families
to adjust to. It is easy for rehabilitation staff, who never knew the person
before the injury, to simply see a 'difficult' or 'aggressive' person. There
are particular challenges for nursing and support staff in working with
neurological conditions, particularly if they have had insufficient training in the variety of presentations that they will see clinically. It is vital
that the clinical neuropsychologist works closely with all staff to embed
understanding of the formulation so that the planned intervention is delivered appropriately and effectively.

We have experience of running reflective and professional practice
groups for nursing staff on a regional specialist inpatient neurorehabilitation unit. These groups, which ran for 45 minutes on a fortnightly basis,
were facilitated by the ward psychologists. All nursing staff were invited
to attend, with the exception of the ward sister. The group was confiden-
tial unless participants wished something particular to be fed back to
external parties. The remit of the group, however, was flexible and included space to discuss the challenges faced at work. It quickly emerged
that when patients were admitted to the unit, nurses received no detailed
information regarding diagnosis or prognosis. Handovers were provided
regarding nursing needs, but rarely were they prepared for the cognitive
and behavioural challenges that patients presented with. Unsurprisingly,
they felt undervalued and were not always fully engaged with the rehabilitation programme. As such, the fortnightly sessions soon began to focus
on sharing formulations with them so that they were able to understand
the rationale for particular interventions. At the same time, nursing and
neuropsychology began to meet more frequently to discuss current patients and planned admissions, with a view to aligning treatment plans.
Almost immediately, incidents of challenging behaviour decreased, as
did the number of falls.

This was a simple intervention, but one that required consistent engagement from the psychology team. The group was a protected space
and only functioned as well as it did because the nurses felt valued and
listened to. In this particular example, the psychology team spent time
every day with the nursing team, not simply to discuss clinical issues,
but to find out about staffing levels and to gauge the temperature of the
nursing team working. Feedback indicated that they valued this process

and it impacted positively on patient care. Nursing teams typically make up the largest staff group on wards. They do some of the most physically taxing jobs. But our experience is that they are one of the most neglected parts of the system.

Similarly, it is imperative that all family members are offered substantial brain injury education, ideally over a period of months, particularly as the patient progresses through the 'window of optimum recovery'. It is vital to remember that the families of those who have sustained severe brain injuries may have frequently felt as though they had been 'lied to' by treating teams. Immediately following the injury, many are told that their loved one will not survive. If they do survive, families may be told that they will never emerge from a coma and, if they do, they will never recognise their family members again, or they will never walk again or talk again. But, every time the patient disproves the clinicians – who have, quite understandably, simply been trying to manage expectations – the family system experiences it as the professionals writing the patient off or getting it wrong. Small wonder, then, that by the time the patient is offered specialist rehabilitation, the family's trust in us has been eroded.

This is the context that clinicians must understand. There is no reason for the families of brain injured patients to trust our predictions and, of course, it may not be psychologically safe to trust them. Even if one must trust, family members need to come to terms with the fact that one's life and marriage is irrevocably altered. It cannot be done overnight. So, although clinicians have to manage expectations, and although our tendency is likely to be cautious at best and pessimistic at worst, we must keep in mind what families need. Clear clinical opinions delivered gently, bearing in mind what the system can tolerate, are the optimum. There is often a tendency for treating teams to demand that the familial systems 'gain some insight' into the reality of the situation. We consider this a somewhat arrogant position to hold. It is unlikely that the spouse of a person with a severe brain injury is unable to consider the reality of the situation, but it is highly likely that their limbic system is activated and they are feeling threatened. A reframe of this kind might help us to work with them more effectively.

At its heart, humility is about upskilling those we work with, whether colleagues or the familial system. The neuropsychologist may hold significant knowledge, but the democratisation of that knowledge is vital. A formulation kept in a filing cabinet is no good; only a formulation shared with the system can lead to effective intervention. Mental capacity assessments are vital, but the Best Interests process can only be effective if all parties understand the principles and the rationale for clinical decision-making. Behavioural management plans are useless if those people implementing them – usually the people with the least specialist training – do not understand them. The good neuropsychologist will be the useful one – the one who is able to understand this, work with the system, and help in the most clinically appropriate way.

Supervision

Clinical Psychology courses, which are typically between two and four days in length, provide supervisor training for local qualified psychologists. It is a requirement to complete this training only if supervising trainee psychologists, not for the supervision of other members of staff. Neuropsychology is a distinct discipline and requires supporting supervisees with specific skills, such as differential diagnosis and neuropsychological assessment, formulation, and intervention. A survey conducted in the US indicated that only 27% of respondents practicing neuropsychology received specific neuropsychological supervision training, with many reporting that they felt inadequately trained (Schultz et al., 2014). The context of neuropsychology in the UK is different from the US, yet there is similarity in that there is no neuropsychology-specific supervision training. The belief that experience alone renders clinicians competent to supervise embodies the antithesis of humility and can be detrimental to patient care and supervisees.

The Qualification in Clinical Neuropsychology (QICN) is seen as the gold standard for demonstrating competency as a clinical neuropsychologist in the UK. The pathway to QICN relies heavily on supervision to support candidates, with a minimum of 60 hours of supervised practice as standard required over a two-year, full-time-equivalent period. Historically, the British Psychological Society route was the only option to become registered as a neuropsychologist, but now the University of Glasgow, University of Bristol, and Salomons Institute offer structured pathways to support candidates to be eligible for entry onto the Specialist Register for Neuropsychologists (SRCN). These developments indicate with even more pertinence the need for supervisors to be aware of course-specific requirements and to have further training to be able to guide candidates successfully.

Neuropsychology supervision routinely involves functional core competencies. This includes knowledge; performance of particular skills, such as assessment, differential diagnosis, and producing specific work, such as reports; as well as providing feedback and intervention (Gates & Sendiack, 2020). However, this approach can fail to facilitate the development of foundational competencies, which include reflective practice, personal awareness, resilience, relationships, interdisciplinary systems, and individual and cultural diversity. Humility could present an opportunity to develop these competencies.

Three types of humility have been indicated within the supervisory context: relational, cultural, and intellectual (Watkins et al., 2019). Relational humility in supervision refers to supervisors being able to foster a good relationship. This includes honesty, openness, responsiveness to feedback, taking responsibility, apologising for mistakes, and taking action to repair ruptures.

Culturally humble supervisors champion a culturally self-aware perspective and attitude of cultural respect. In practice, this means not shying away from having conversations in relation to individual differences and thinking about this meaningfully with regards to the relationship, the wider team, and the clinical work. This is particularly important when supporting supervisees to develop a critical understanding of the role of neuropsychology and how this is applied in different communities. Of course, supervision is not therapy, and that boundary should be respected. However, a supervisor taking the time to get to know their supervisee can help to contextualise their needs and guide how to support them in their work and the workplace. Microaggressions, which are the everyday, subtle, intentional, and sometimes unintentional interactions or behaviours that communicate bias toward historically marginalized groups (DeAngelis, 2009), are more likely to occur when supervisors fail to demonstrate cultural humility.

Intellectual humility involves the balance between neither overvaluing nor undervaluing intellectual ability (Church & Barrett, 2016). It involves understanding intellectual limitations and a desire to be informed by the opinions of others. In the neuropsychology supervisory context, an example could be supporting supervisees to find their own style in their work. However, less experienced clinicians, who initially need more direction, structure, and concrete guidance, could perceive an expression of supervisor humility as reflecting a lack of supervisory containment or competence (McNeill & Stoltenberg, 2016).

Humility is a useful quality for both the supervisor and supervisee to foster in the supervisory relationship and could aid the development of foundational competencies. The focus in this section has been on supervisor humility because, ultimately, the supervisor holds considerable power in the relationship. In practice, a 'good enough' blend of the different types of humility would be the ideal to aim for, with some situations or supervisory relationships requiring more of one type of humility over another. Good supervision practices are also important, such as the use of supervision contracts to negotiate and outline the structure and respective responsibilities and the use of good, mutually shared note keeping. These practices can be a good way to build a foundation of psychological safety, as it creates a point to return to for renegotiating the relationship when there are ruptures or facilitating periodic reviews of supervision. The humility to seek and respond to feedback is the cornerstone of a humble supervisor.

Teaching and Research

A fundamental oversight in clinical psychology doctorate courses is the explicit explanation that neuropsychology and biology are fundamental in every specialty of clinical psychology. A common conundrum that clinical psychologists and neuropsychologists face is teasing out whether someone presenting for support is displaying mental health difficulties, some undiagnosed neurodiversity, some other neurological condition, or some combination of all of the above. The failure to adequately embed neuropsychology throughout the whole of clinical psychology training means we contribute to the gaps between services that patients with co-morbid needs can fall into. Furthermore, the lack of overlap between paediatric neuropsychology and adult neuropsychology is another area in which skills, resources, and knowledge are lost.

Clinical psychologists working in a non-neurological specialty may accurately assess that they do not know enough about neuropsychology and, therefore, they avoid clinical tasks they associate with it. This may include evading cognitive assessments that might compliment information in the formulation or lacking the confidence or awareness to ask questions as part of the clinical assessment to make sense of a patient's brain health. From the perspective of humility, this captures being aware of the limits of knowledge. However, it but does not capture the intentionality in taking responsibility for continuous learning and development to address these gaps in knowledge. Equally, the same can be said of clinical neuropsychologists who have worked for years in very specialist areas of neuropsychology and who have possibly become deskilled around mental health more broadly. Beyond the scope of training and individual clinician self-awareness, this problem also highlights the need for consultancy and supervision between psychologists across specialties to share knowledge and skills.

The manner in which teaching is approached during clinical psychology training and in post-qualification neuropsychology courses appears to lack the involvement of people with neurological conditions. It speaks to an absence of intellectual humility that there is scarcity in co-production and collaboration with the people we are being trained to provide services for. When people with neurological conditions are invited to participate in teaching, it is all too often reduced to a short time slot when they are invited to share their experience of living with a neurological condition. Whilst this contribution is much valued when it is included, it reinforces unhelpful power dynamics regarding professional and patient relationships.

Humility in research can also be of great benefit. In considering a research question, it is important to consider whether unhelpful stereotypes about particular neurological conditions or communities are being reinforced. When considering the sample used in research studies, it is important to consider the demographics represented and what this means for generalisability. Ray et al. (2022) found that Black communities remain disproportionately under-represented in neuropsychology research. This study was focused on research in US, so it remains unknown what the picture is like in the UK context. However, given the challenges NHS services face regarding being inclusive to communities from racially minoritized communities, it seems likely to be a similar area of concern. There are noted disparities in health based on gender, sexuality, race, and social class linked to a range of structural inequalities and social determinants of health. As a result, it is important that cultural humility is exercised in the design, recruitment, reporting, and dissemination of research. This is particularly important for intervention research so we can ensure that the data we use to guide 'best practice' is inclusive of a range of communities.

Conclusion: Where Next for Humility in Neuropsychology?

It is by no means easy to consistently embody humility. It requires purposeful action to adopt this quality in all that we do professionally. It serves no one for clinical neuropsychologists to diminish what they can offer. However, humility will require us to climb down from our ivory towers to reduce power differentials, take a systemic approach, and really understand what it is for patients to have significant unmet social needs. The adoption of a 'common language' can result in improvement of assessment, treatment, as well as staff and patient experiences. There is also a need to work across psychology specialties to share resources and knowledge as part of a mutually beneficial skill exchange.

It is often said that to know where you are going you have to know where you have come from. Therefore, an understanding of the history of neuropsychology that accurately reflects the historical socio-political impact is a necessity. Knowing our history means being able to do things differently, as short memories lead to repeated attempts to implement the same solutions and the stifling of innovation. We must never lose sight of the fact that, broadly speaking, the paradigms of understanding we embrace today will inevitably shift at some point in the future. There is seldom one right way or answer, and we have to keep learning, reflecting, and evolving. The COVID pandemic moved neuropsychology rapidly ahead of where we would otherwise be because it forced us to let go of rigid beliefs about how we practice and reluctantly embrace changes which were long resisted but hard fought for. In lieu of another pandemic or mass global event that forces us to adapt further, the standard of how we practice needs to embody openness, willingness, collaboration, and, fundamentally, humility.

References

Annon, J. (1976). The PLISSIT model: A proposed conceptual scheme for the behavioural treatment of sexual problems. *Journal of Sex Education and Therapy*, *2*, 1–15. DOI: 10.1080/01614576.1976.11074483.

Barnett, W. S. (1998). Long-term cognitive and academic effects of early childhood education on children in poverty. *Preventive Medicine*, *27*(2), 204–207.

British Psychological Society. (2007). *Leading Psychological Services.* British Psychological Society. https://www.bps.org.uk/sites/www.bps.org.uk/files/Member%20Networks/Faculties/Leadership/Leading%20Psychological%20Services%20A%20report%20by%20the%20Division%20of%20Clinical%20Psychology%20-%20BPS%20%282007%29.pdf.

Calabrò, R. S., & Bramanti, P. (2014). Post-stroke sexual dysfunction: An overlooked and under-addressed problem. *Disability and Rehabilitation, 36*(3): 263–264. DOI: 10.3109/09638288.2013.785603.

Casaletto, K. B., & Heaton, R. K. (2017). Neuropsychological assessment: Past and future. *Journal of the International Neuropsychological Society, 23*(9–10), 778–790.

Church, I., & Barrett, J. (2016). Intellectual Humility. In E. L. Worthington Jr., D. E. Davis, & J. N. Hook (Eds.) *Handbook of Humility: Theory, Research, and Applications* (pp. 62–75). Routledge.

Coard, B. (1971). Making black children subnormal in Britain. *Integrated Education: Race and Schools, 9*(5), 49–52.

Colman, A. M. (2016). Race differences in IQ: Hans Eysenck's contribution to the debate in the light of subsequent research. *Personality and Individual Differences, 103*, 182–189.

DeAngelis, T. (2009). Unmasking 'racial micro aggressions.' *American Psychological Association: Monitor on Psychology, 40*(2), 42.

Del Re, A. C., Flückiger, C., Horvath, A. O., Symonds, D., & Wampold, B. E. (2012). Therapist effects in the therapeutic alliance-outcome relationship: A restricted-maximum likelihood meta-analysis. *Clinical Psychology Review, 32*, 642–649.

Eells, T. D. (1997). *Handbook of psychotherapy case formulation.* Guilford Press.

Eysenck, H. J. (1971). *The IQ Argument: Race, Intelligence and Education.* Library Press.

Gates, N. J., & Sendiack, C. L. (2017). Neuropsychology Supervision: Incorporating Reflective Practice, Australian Psychologist, *52*(3), 191–197. DOI: 10.1111/ap.12242.

Huynh, H. P., & Dicke-Bohmann, A. (2020). Humble doctors, healthy patients?: Exploring the relationships between clinician humility and patient satisfaction, trust, and health status. *Patient Education and Counseling, 103*(1), 173–179.

Macniven, J. A. B. (2015). *Neuropsychological formulation: A clinical casebook.* Springer.

McNeill, B. W., & Stoltenberg, C. D. (2016). *Supervision essentials for the integrative developmental model.* American Psychological Association. DOI: 10.1037/14858-000.

Nell, V. (1999). *Cross-cultural neuropsychological assessment: Theory and practice.* Psychology Press.

Norrgard, K. (2008). Human testing, the eugenics movement, and IRBs. *Nature Education, 1*(1), 170.

Owen, J., Tao, K. W., Drinane, J. M., Hook, J., Davis, D. E., & Kune, N. F. (2016). Client perceptions of therapists' multicultural orientation: Cultural (missed) opportunities and cultural humility. *Professional Psychology: Research and Practice, 47*(1), 30–37. DOI: 10.1037/pro0000046.

Plato. (1871). *Laches or Courage.* Trans. B. Jowett. Scribner's Sons. Retrieved from https://www.sacred-texts.com/cla/plato/laches.htm. (Original work published 380 BC).

Ray, C. G. L., Mariouw, K. H., Anderson, K. M., George, E., Bisignano, N., Hernandez, S., & Montgomery, V. L. (2022). Current status of inclusion of black subjects in neuropsychological studies: A scoping review and call to action. *Clinical Neuropsychologist, 36*(2), 227–244. DOI: 10.1080/13854046.2021.2019314.

Richards, A., Dean, R., Burgess, G. H., & Caird, H. (2016). Sexuality after stroke: An exploration of current professional approaches, barriers to providing support and future directions. *Disability and Rehabilitation, 38*(15), 1471–1482. DOI: 10.3109/09638288.2015.1106595.

Rudd, A. G., Bowen, A., Young, G. R., & James, M. A. (2017). The latest national clinical guideline for stroke. *Clinical Medicine, 17*(2), 154–155. DOI: 10.7861/clinmedicine.17-2-154.

Sariaslan, A., Sharp, D. J., D'Onofrio, B. M., Larsson, H., & Fazel, S. (2016). Long-term outcomes associated with traumatic brain injury in childhood and adolescence: A nationwide Swedish cohort study of a wide range of medical and social outcomes. *PLoS medicine, 13*(8), e1002103.

Schmidt, N. B., & Woolaway-Bickel, K. (2000). The effects of treatment compliance on outcome in cognitive-behavioral therapy for panic disorder: Quality versus quantity. *Journal of Consulting and Clinical Psychology, 68*, 13–18.

Schultz, L. A., Pedersen, H. A., Roper, B. L., & Rey-Casserly, C. (2014). Supervision in neuropsychological assessment: A survey of training, practice, and perspectives of supervisors. *Clinical Neuropsychologist, 28*(6), 907–925. DOI: 10.1080/13854046.2014.942373

Smail, D. J. (2005). *Power, Interest and Psychology: Elements of a social materialist understanding of distress.* PCCS Books.

Spencer, J., Goode, J., Penix, E. A., Trusty, W., & Swift, J. K. (2019). Developing a collaborative relationship with clients during the initial sessions of psychotherapy. *Psychotherapy, 56*(1), 7–10.

Stein, J., Hillinger, M., Clancy, C., & Bishop, L. (2013). Sexuality after stroke: Patient counseling preferences. *Disability and Rehabilitation, 35*(21), 1842–1847. DOI: 10.3109/09638288.2012.754953.

Templeton, J. M. (1997). *Worldwide laws of life.* Templeton Foundation Press

Tervalon, M., & Murray-García, J. (1998). Cultural humility versus cultural competence: A critical distinction in defining physician training outcomes in multicultural education. *Journal of Health Care for the Poor and Underserved, 9*(2), 117–125.

Wagner, E. H., Bennett, S. M., Austin, B. T., Greene, S. M., Schaefer, J. K., & Vonkorff, M. (2005). Finding common ground: Patient-centeredness and evidence-based chronic illness care. *Journal of Alternative and Complementary Medicine, 11*(1), S7–15. DOI: 10.1089/acm.2005.11.s-7.

Watkins, E., Hook, J. N., Mosher, D. K., & Callahan, J. L. (2019). Humility in clinical supervision: Fundamental, foundational, and transformational. *The Clinical Supervisor, 38*(1), 58–78, DOI: 10.1080/07325223.2018.1487355.

Whiffin, C. J., Gracey, F., & Ellis-Hill, C. (2021). The experience of families following traumatic brain injury in adult populations: A meta-synthesis of narrative structures. *International Journal of Nursing Studies, 123*, 104043. DOI: 10.1016/j.ijnurstu.2021.104043.

Yang, J., Zhang, W., & Chen, X. (2019). Why do leaders express humility and how does this matter: a rational choice perspective? *Frontiers in Psychology, 10*, 19–25.

12 Leading Neuropsychology Services in the 21st Century

Deconstructing Leadership

Amanda Mobley

Introduction: What Do We Mean by Leadership?

After a period of maternity leave, I returned to a team I had been working in for a number of years. When I left the team had been thriving and resilient, yet when I returned the team appeared low in energy with brewing conflicts between professionals. This was not for lack of innovative and committed staff. So, what had changed in this time? The team lead had left. The lead had guided the team with good humour and authentic trust through a number of difficult years. Without this presence the team felt disjointed, lost, and drifting. This is difference authentic leadership can make: it does not necessarily change the context, but it can enable people to work in the face of adversity.

Authentic leadership 'draws upon and promotes both positive psychological capacities and a positive ethical climate, to foster greater self-awareness, an internalized moral perspective, balanced processing of information, and relational transparency' (Walumbwa et al., 2008, p. 94). For the purposes of this chapter, I use this definition to incorporate leadership of services as well as professional or project leadership.

In recognising systemic influence, I wanted to reference my own personal context. I am a White, heterosexual, cisgendered woman, and I'm approaching leadership from the experience of primarily working in the NHS. In my current role, I am the head of a moderately large neuropsychology department covering a rich, diverse urban and rural community. As a clinician and leader, I have always been drawn to relational approaches and the potential such approaches build for change and growth. My intention is that this chapter will draw out ways of developing these conversations and provide a structure for ongoing dialogue about diversity within neuropsychology. I make particular reference to White privilege, but this could be conceived as privilege within other domains. I have intentionally used the language of 'we' or 'I' to make it clear that this is my experience/position and does not mean to imply a universal truth.

DOI: 10.4324/9781003309819-16

What Are the Current Issues Facing Leaders in Neuropsychology?

The Black Lives Matter movement and the COVID-19 pandemic have highlighted long-standing and previously ignored institutional discrimination within the UK. Healthcare research has shown that ethnic-minority communities in the UK experience barriers to accessing to services, poorer experience of services, and reduction in expected outcomes relative to their White counterparts (Kapadia et al, 2022). This is despite people from minoritised communities often having more socio-economic stressors and associated health concerns. Key authors (e.g., Rivera Mindt et al., 2010) have been researching cross-cultural neuropsychology and institutional discrimination in neuropsychology for a number of years, highlighting, for example, the Eurocentric/Western nature of most standard neuropsychological batteries. However, neuropsychology as a profession is only at the start of its journey of recognising the impact of White privilege and the wide-reaching ramifications on service users, families, professionals, and policymakers. In addition to this, it is becoming clear that COVID-19 has had a disproportionate effect on people with neurological conditions, especially those from ethnic minorities, who may have faced lengthy isolation from family whilst in hospital, experienced expedited discharge, received reduced rehabilitation input, and tolerated delayed appointments, to name a few areas of concern (Neurological Alliance, 2020).

Why Systemic Approaches in Leadership?

At its heart, leadership implies there are people or there is a project that requires guidance, support, and/or decision-making. As such, leadership is fundamentally relational in nature, and a leader cannot exist independently of the team, project, or policy on which they are leading. Indeed, the relationships between the leader and members of the team are often the very mechanism of change. The process comes down to how well a leader works with these relationships to produce effective change. Lang, Little, and Cronen (1990) propose that, in order to balance the need for decision-making with collaboration, clinicians can work between domains of *production* (taking action) and *explanation* (exploring the range of possibilities), while leaders need an *aesthetic* domain to decide when and how to move between production and explanation. In this respect, systemic approaches can provide a highly practical framework to understand the balance required in leadership.

Systemic approaches are fundamentally concerned with discourse and opening up conversations as a way of creating 'the difference that makes the difference'. I often find myself particularly drawn to narrative approaches to provide insights in leadership and diversity. The narrative approach can be described as working with the stories people tell about their lives, while recognising people as distinct from the problems they experience and as having a range of strengths and resources from which to draw (White & Epston, 1990).

The Role of Context

Leaders do not exist within a vacuum. They are subject to the pressures of the service/project, and they bring their own cultural, occupational, and personal context. Burnham's (2013) Social GGRRAAACCEEESSS model can facilitate leaders to be reflexive of their own stories and lived experience as well as draw attention to their blind spots and unconscious biases. There has been some critique of this model for being reductionist to a list of characteristics (Birdsey & Kustner, 2020), and approaches such as intersectionality (Crenshaw, 1989) can help leaders to recognise the mutual influences these characteristics may have on one another. Leaders need to take time to recognise the power and privilege associated with these characteristics, for example, unpacking the invisible knapsack of privilege in neuropsychology, as aptly demonstrated by Cory (2021). For my part, recognising this context has drawn my attention to the unearned benefits of being White in the world of neuropsychology.

Leaders have an invitation to recognise the roles their staff members have beyond their work role, and this places leaders in a unique position to either sustain or transform the status quo. Asking questions such as: Are the staff within the service culturally representative of the community they serve? How accessible is the service/profession for people from diverse backgrounds? What is the role and impact of micro-aggressions or allyship on the working life of staff? How do staff members feel if their cultural heritage is not represented within the profession as whole or at senior leadership levels? This has additional relevance in neuropsychology, as staff may be working with people with brain injuries who possibly, as a consequence of executive dysfunction, may overtly subject staff to prejudice and discrimination. For example, how does a leader support the team working with a person with a brain injury who requires rehabilitation but is subjecting staff from ethnic minorities to racial discrimination and abuse?

Furthermore, each service, project, or policy has a rich and detailed history that has led to its creation and intersections within the system. For example, how and why was a service first created? Who has led the service in the past, and whose views have shaped how the service was delivered, funded, and operationalised? How does the service relate to other services/projects and the community it serves? For example, a service that has been under-resourced, and therefore has had to narrow referral criteria, may be seen as inaccessible. This has the potential to disproportionately affect those who need more bespoke assessment, such as those from non-Western cultural backgrounds, where a standard assessment protocol may not be suitable. This may lead clinicians to either reject a referral as too complex or administer an assessment which does not meet the individual's needs. Asking questions which seek to understand both the history and context of a service can enable leaders to reflexively engage with this context and set out their hopes and intentions for the future.

Language as a Mechanism of Change

The use of language is critical because systemic practice is typically rooted in a social-constructionist understanding of the world, whereby assumptions and knowledge about the world are co-created between people. Language is the vehicle for this construction, so use of language in leadership is key. Language can also be an avenue for microaggressions, creating a context of 'otherness' and stigmatisation of difference, whether this be towards staff members or service users, and so warrants further attention of those in positions of leadership.

Language shapes expectations for service users and staff alike, for example, consider service information leaflets. Service information leaflets are typically couched in 'professional' language about different roles and what is offered. This presumes socialisation with the medical model and individual model of rehabilitation; whereas, in practice, the meaning of these terms can have different implications within different communities. Subsequently, terms such as *post-traumatic amnesia* or *dementia* can be misunderstood or confused. This is crucial because the language of the information leaflet shapes the expectations of new or potential staff and service users, even before the first contact with a service.

Through this same mechanism, however, language allows us the opportunity, space, and potential to provide transformational leadership. Language offers the opportunity to reframe or acknowledge conflicting views. Language enables us to express ourselves as leaders and show our individuality and values through the words that we choose. Ultimately, language gives us the chance to reflect on how we ask questions and, as discussed later on, the use of narratives gives us a chance to think about who is being asked and who is answering.

Externalisation and using language to construct 'the problem as the problem rather than people as the problem' (White & Epston, 1990) can enable leaders to understand when teams or projects are stuck, for example, 'the whiteness of neuropsychology'. The process of externalisation: naming/characterising the problem, considering the effects of the problem, and looking at positions on the problem and the values underpinning each position can facilitate joint conversations without blame being located within one party or another. This 'de-centering' creates space between the 'people' involved and the 'problem' they are trying to solve. As such, this can work towards an approach from a position of togetherness, problem-solving, and curiosity. When policymakers and teams recognise they are all in a relationship with the problem, such as the Whiteness of neuropsychology, then they can see there are various alternative positions that can be taken to help promote change.

Narratives

Leadership, in the domain of production, requires taking action. In order to take action appropriately, leaders need to attend to the domain of explanation and explore the multiverse of ideas to ensure all voices are heard. Leaders need to remain aware of whose voice is being heard, whose voice is being prioritised, and notice 'thin' narratives. A thin narrative privileges one story over the multiplicity, and inflexible narratives can lead to defined, rigid responses. This defined set of responses then affects how staff teams or individuals engage with both current and future events. Dominant thin narratives are shaped by the context and the language being used, for example, narratives within neuropsychology about sticking with existing test batteries and norms even in the face of evidence that this is not suitable for a large number of our service users.

Systemic aspects of leadership enable us to consider what the unheard aspects of this narrative might be, what are the areas of strength or the stories of success that have been deprioritised, and how do we strengthen these narratives to provide a holistic and balanced view. For example, clinicians have made headway in developing alternative methods of assessment. The role of the leader, as in therapy, is not necessarily to dismantle a narrative but to develop a richer and more nuanced holistic view, which encompasses challenges and hardship as well as strengths and values. Skill in drawing out narratives also assists in recognising those narratives that have not been heard. Within our service, as in many services, we have a satisfaction questionnaire which takes the form of a range of scaled and yes/no questions. However, does this facilitate feedback from everyone? Does this respect different ways of communicating for those who prefer to give feedback in a verbal form or in a group setting? So, by using a questionnaire method, whose voices are being prioritised, and how does this shape the direction of the service?

To consider narratives is also to consider power and the role that power plays in neuropsychology. The power associated with leadership provides challenges and opportunities at the same time. Leaders have a role in shaping and scaffolding who gets to tell their story and how and where that story is heard. This also means that leaders have a unique opportunity to make a reflective space for this discussion and examination of who holds power and how this is used.

This links with positioning theory and both how people position themselves and how they are positioned by others/society (van Langenhove &

Harré, 1999). Positions are a relational space in comparison with other people, for example, this may be birth order relative to siblings or expertise relative to members of the public. The positions people take come with a pre-existing set of expectations and behaviours. For example, dominant narratives within society typically give greater emphasis to the expertise of a professional over the role of lived experience. As such, the role of professional comes with a set of expectations, such as the individual is able to give an expert opinion or categorically answer a question (Hare-Mustin, 1994). The impact of these expectations is evident in recruitment practices, where experience as a volunteer assistant psychologist is often accorded more credit than lived experiences. In line with this thinking, leaders are frequently accorded greater authority than other members of a team, and this can have an interactive effect with White privilege. If a leader is consciously aware of taking or being put in this position, then they are able to open up conversations about alternative positions which they might take. This is not about having a desired 'end point' but giving space to develop and thicken alternative narratives, build flexibility, and recognise exceptions. This may then pave the way to reflect on how services are positioned by minoritised communities and work towards creating more equitable services.

Narratives also give an avenue for 'systemic justice' and encouraging discourse on Human Rights, for example, the Dulwich Centre Charter on Story-Telling Rights (Denborough, 2014). Encouraging service users and people with neurological conditions to tell their stories as the basis for policy and political change can be seen in the work of the All-Party Parliamentary Groups (APPGs). People with neurological conditions can often have unheard stories within wider society, for example, when individuals do not externally appear unwell and their difficulties are minimised, or when people with more severe brain injuries are reliant on others to help them to express their stories. However, this can intersect with narratives around privilege and consideration of how many within those service users with brain injury and neurological conditions who influence policy are from ethnic minorities.

Strengths and Resources: An Appreciative Stance

Systemic approaches also highlight the role of the strengths and resources people have in their lives. These strengths might be exceptions from the dominant narrative approaches, and a leader can 'double listen' for these stories of hope or strength in addition to listening to stories of 'stuckness' or loss (Guilfoyle, 2014). Even the act of witnessing or noticing the hope or the dignity with which an individual has responded can change a conversation (Wade, 1997).

Within many health contexts, we often speak in terms of 'barriers', and neuropsychology is no exception. In a national mapping survey questionnaire, we initially started trying to understand the 'barriers' to accessing neuropsychology services. However, where does this take the narrative, and what does this enable us to do with this information? We are acutely aware of dominant narratives of long wait times for services and the challenges of under-resourced staffing. Consequently, we reframed this to ask about contexts in which services had worked well with the intention of attending to stories of resilience and building on existing innovation, paying attention not just to staff numbers, but to diversity within the neuropsychology staff workforce.

Systems and organisations need difference to drive innovation, and one of the challenges of systemic practice can be balancing the need for difference and the need for finding a common ground. When leaders have established an understanding of and respect for the differences in context, narratives, and strengths, then they can work towards establishing the commonalities, for example, everyone wants to work towards anti-discriminatory practice.

Transparency and Authenticity

Core principles of any systemic approach are transparency and asking questions to which you genuinely do not know the answers. Genuine transparency challenges leaders to probe their beliefs, inherent assumptions, and biases in a curious and self-reflexive way (Rober, 2005). This can then facilitate collaboration and co-production as it recognises the gaps in knowledge and necessitates seeking the knowledge and skills of others to support these. However, this can also be confronting to the sense of the 'professional self' as this requires leaders to be vulnerable, take relational risks, and bring themselves to the leadership role. Despite this, my experience has been that bringing the 'self' into leadership also permits others to do this. I often start a meeting with an honest reflection of where I am that day – if I have been stuck in traffic, I had a bad night with my children, or I lack certainty about a solution for a topic we are discussing, such as, how we support equitable access, experience, and outcomes for all who encounter our neuropsychology service. My intention is that this enables people to feel that their 'selves' are important and recognised as individuals with their own contexts.

Mason (1993) offers a framework of 'safe uncertainty' based along axes of safety and certainty. In order to explore the available possibilities, leaders need to create a position of 'safe uncertainty' through inquiry from 'authoritative doubt'. Mason highlights there is rarely one ultimate solution, as each solution may raise new dilemmas. This moves us towards a position of sitting with and explicitly acknowledging uncertainty whilst simultaneously opening up space for new possibilities through mutual influence and respectful curiosity.

Lifecycles and Transitions

Within systemic theory, lifecycle transition points, such as births or deaths, can raise key challenges but can also open up conversations that otherwise might not have been able to happen. These lifecycles and multi-generational conversations also occur in our professional lives through the lifecycles of the people, structures, and ideas. Any transition or change can be highly unsettling for all involved, as existing narratives, whether these be helpful or unhelpful, can provide a sense of continuity and stability. If we consider the impact of the death of George Floyd and the Black Lives Matter protests around the world, we can consider how this has influenced neuropsychology and the challenges of holding the discomfort provoked by this. And yet, arguably this has enabled a substantial shift in the conversation within the profession. This has led to discussions about White privilege, such as, whether neuropsychological assessment is or can be culturally fair, whether there are alternative collectivist or community models of rehabilitation to complement or sit alongside an individual model, and how to increase the richness and diversity within the profession.

Transition and lifecycles can also apply to ideas and the recruitment and teaching of new 'generations' of professionals. There is a growing awareness that, without reflection and insight into unconscious bias, there is a risk that these cycles facilitate existing privileges. However, these lifecycles can be an opportunity for leaders to speak to the discourses of power that underpin the profession, especially those pertaining to diversity. In this way, leaders have a role not only in shaping the current narrative but also the transition to future narratives.

Conclusion: What Now?

To bring this chapter to a close and to consider 'What now?' for systemic leadership in neuropsychology, I wanted to reflect on the key points and pose some reflective questions:

- Leadership is inherently relational in nature, so systemic approaches may be useful to help understand our role as leaders.
- There are benefits to leaders understanding and respecting the social, political, cultural, and historical context of a service or project.
- How do we reflect on language and the use of language as a fundamental aspect of leadership?
- In what ways can leaders in neuropsychology consider the stories that are told, who gets to tell their story, and whose voices are not heard? How do leaders support all voices to be heard and promote a collaborative approach?
- How can leaders orient towards strengths and resources within a system using self-reflexivity and reflective practice in neuropsychology?

- In what ways can be bring our authentic selves to leadership roles and create a context of safe uncertainty?
- How do we respect and reflect on lifecycles within a professional life-cycle sphere, the role of privilege, and the opportunities that these transition points can represent?
- How might leaders facilitate or create the context for the development and embedment of systemic skills in neuropsychology?

References

Birdsey, N., & Kustner, C. (2020). Reviewing the Social GRACES: What Do They Add and Limit in Systemic Thinking and Practice? *American Journal of Family Therapy, 49*(2), 429–442. DOI: 10.1080/01926187.2020.1830731.

Burnham, J. (2013). *Developments in Social GGRRAAACCEEESSS: Visible-invisible and voiced-unvoiced.* In I.-B. Krause (Ed.), *Culture and Reflexivity in Systemic Psychotherapy* (pp. 139–160). Routledge.

Cory, J. M. (2021). White privilege in neuropsychology: An 'invisible knapsack' in need of unpacking? *The Clinical Neuropsychologist, 35*(2), 206–218.

Crenshaw, K. W. (1989). Demarginalising the intersection of race and sex: A black feminist critique of antidiscrimination doctrine, feminist theory and antiracist politics. *University of Chicago Legal Forum, 140*(1), 139–167.

Denborough, D. (2014). *Retelling the Stories of Our Lives: Everyday Narrative Therapy to Draw Inspiration and Transform Experience.* W. W. Norton.

Guilfoyle, M. (2014). Listening in narrative therapy: Double listening and empathic positioning. *South African Journal of Psychology, 45*(1), 36–49.

Hare-Mustin, R. (1994). Discourses in the Mirrored Room: A Postmoden Analysis of Therapy, *Family Process*, 33, 19–35.

Kapadia, D., Zhang, J., Salway, S., Nazroo, J., Booth, A., Villarroel-Williams, N., Becares, L., & Esmail, A. (2022). *Ethnic Inequalities in Healthcare: A Rapid Evidence Review.* NHS Race & Health Observatory.

Lang, P., Little, M., & Cronen, V. (1990). The Systemic Professional: Domains of Action and the Question of Neutrality. *Human Systems: The Journal of Systemic Consultation and Management, 1*, 32–47.

Mason, B. (1993). Towards positions of safe uncertainty. *Human Systems, 3*(3–4), 189–200.

Neurological Alliance. (2020). *Restarting services for people with neurological conditions after the COVID-19 pandemic and planning for the longer term.* The Neurological Alliance.

Rivera Mindt, M., Byrd, D., Saez, P., & Manly, J. (2010). Increasing culturally competent neuropsychological services for ethnic minority populations: A call to action. *Clinical Neuropsychology, 24*(3): 429–453. DOI: 10.1080/13854040903058960.

Rober, P. (2005). The therapist's self in dialogical family therapy: Some ideas about not-knowing and the therapists inner conversation. *Family Process, 44*(4), 477–495.

van Langenhove, L., & Harré, R. (1999). Introducing positioning theory. In R. Harré & L. van Langenhove (Eds.), *Positioning Theory* (pp. 14–31). Blackwell.

Wade, A. (1997). Small acts of living: Everyday resistance to violence and other forms of oppression. *Contemporary Family Therapy*, 19*(1)*, 23–39.

Walumbwa, F. O., Avolio, B. J., Gardner, W. L., Wernsing, T. S., & Peterson, S. J. (2008). Authentic leadership: Development and validation of a theory-based measure. *Journal of Management*, *34*, 89–126.

White, M., & Epston, D. (1990). *Narrative Means to Therapeutic Ends*. W. W. Norton.

Part 5
Moving Forward

13 Workforce

Inclusion in Clinical Neuropsychology

Carol Sampson

Introduction

Clinical neuropsychology services are increasingly delivered through a broad range of organisations. As well as the NHS, other stakeholders include social care organisations, education establishments, and community organisations (Palmer et al., 2021; Rachel, 2011). In an increasingly diverse society, there is also a need to consider cultural influences and socioeconomic dynamics in the interactions between service users and neuropsychologists. In addition, the importance of reducing our own biases within the therapeutic space has been highlighted by Hays (2016). The ADDRESSING model introduced by Hays (2016) provides a framework for helping professionals to self-reflect on the biases and values embedded in their own cultural identity.

National Drivers for Changes to the Neuropsychology Workforce

To determine the enablers and barriers to the development of multicultural neuropsychology (as described in Chapter 1), an awareness of national policies and recommendations is useful. The NHS Workforce Race Equality Standard (2020) documents the need to counter significant discriminatory processes impacting on the selection, recruitment, and retention of staff from minority ethnic groups. Recommendations for addressing these issues and instigating change at the organisational level have been proposed by Kline (2021) and Ross et al., (2020) for example, by having clear leadership and changing the work climate and organisational context. Kapadia et al. (2022) also reviewed research on the experiences of NHS healthcare workers from various ethnic minoritised groups. Findings include high levels of discrimination experienced by Black African nurses from White British nurses, patients, and managers (Likupe et al., 2013). Asian and Black healthcare staff were also more likely to report experiencing discrimination compared to White staff (Rhead et al., 2021).

Our current psychological professions workforce is under-representative of ethnic minorities, people with disabilities, and men, and it is increasingly

DOI: 10.4324/9781003309819-18

skewed towards youth (Health Education England, 2021). There are relatively few studies on the ethnic makeup of the UK clinical neuropsychology workforce and if this reflects the populations served at the local level (Baber, 2020). More consistent workforce data collection is needed to determine the full impact of the relationship between ethnic diversity and effectiveness of clinical neuropsychology service provision in the UK.

At a national level, the British Psychological Society (BPS) established the Equality, Diversity, and Inclusion (EDI) Taskforce with the aim of translating the Society's stated commitment to valuing diversity and promoting inclusion into concrete actions (BPS, 2020). The BPS has recently announced a plan to consolidate the work of the taskforce by developing an EDI strategic board as part of the senior organisational structure (BPS, 2021).

Recognition of the need to address EDI issues in a systematic way has also led to several BPS divisions setting up EDI structures. The Division of Neuropsychology EDI group has developed resources relating to the support and promotion of a more ethnically inclusive profession within the context of developing workstreams on a broader range of protected characteristics.

The move towards establishing EDI structures within the BPS is not without its critics. Ahsan (2022) challenges the idea of EDI work within clinical psychology, referring to it as 'Endless Distraction and Inaction'. Ahsan (2022) focuses on the dangers of the EDI lead as a lone worker within an organisation, pointing out the challenges inherent in calling out existing and embedded structural and institutional racism. Without space for careful planning and resourcing to embed the principles and application of EDI, workstreams within the BPS may also risk becoming marginalised.

The Current Situation within the UK Clinical Neuropsychology Profession

The majority of NHS UK clinical neuropsychologists (60%) work in adult services and have a clinical psychology gateway qualification (Yates, 2017). At the time of the Division of Neuropsychology (DoN) 2017 survey, 72% of the membership was female. There was no data on ethnicity. The lack of data makes it difficult to gain a true reflection of the ethnic make-up of the UK neuropsychology workforce. However, it is known that the majority (84%) of UK clinical psychologists are White and female (Palmer et al., 2021), and this is likely to be similar for the Division of Neuropsychology. The experiences of clinical psychologists from ethnic minoritised backgrounds have been described in several studies. Odusanya et al. (2018) explored the experiences of a group of Black and Asian female clinical psychologists. Several themes emerge from this study, including the need to negotiate personal and professional values (i.e., trying to hold on to cultural identity in the face of incompatible theories and professional ways of being). Also, the idea of 'sitting with uncertainty' was identified to describe the impact of not acknowledging ethnicity in the clinical psychologist and/or client. The findings from this and other research reflect the additional complex layers of being needed by psychologists of colour when interacting in predominantly White spaces.

Barriers and Enablers to Entering the Neuropsychology Workforce

Investment in those aspiring to enter the psychology profession should form a key component of any strategic plan. In recognition of the unique and additional challenges that aspiring psychologists from ethnic minoritised backgrounds face, Health Education England (HEE) (2021) rolled out a programme to fund clinical psychology courses to improve equity and inclusion for Black, Asian, and minority ethnic trainees. This programme is part of the wider HEE psychology workforce development plan (Health Education England, 2021) and includes mentorship development and opportunities to gain relevant employment experience.

Ahsan (2022) shines a critical spotlight on the limitations of the HEE programme and identifies a need to address 'Whiteness' (the systemic processes upholding false hierarchies through rules, norms, and discourses to maintain the so-called superiority of people racialised as White) as a root cause of existing racialised inequalities. This is a powerful assertion that will create discomfort and challenge for some within the profession. Alternatively, it can be seen as an opportunity to further dismantle the structures that have upheld inherent positions of dominance and subjugation and replace them with psychologically healthier alternatives (Nugent, 2019).

Gaining Access to Clinical Neuropsychology Professional Training

When considering the landscape of applied neuropsychology, as noted earlier, clinical psychology is one of the entry gateways. Obtaining entry-level training within clinical psychology is notoriously difficult. Clearing House statistics for 2020 applications indicate that there were 4,225 applicants for 770 places, with only an 18% overall success rate. Nearly 80% of applicants came from a White background (Clearing House, 2021). Palmer et al. (2021) assert that certain minority ethnic groups are less likely to progress in a psychology career than others. Those from Black or Asian ethnic backgrounds going to university are as likely as those with White ethnicity to study psychology and work in NHS psychological professions. However, they are far less likely to be accepted onto a clinical psychology training course and be in more senior NHS roles. Even when successful in gaining entry to the gateway training, clinical psychology trainees from ethnic minoritised backgrounds have reported feelings of alienation, 'unbelonging', and imposter syndrome (Adetimole et al., 2005; Rajan & Shaw, 2008; Onyeama & Yates-Stephenson, 2020).

Community Psychology Approaches

The importance of engaging with service users at the grassroots community level is increasingly recognised. Therefore, psychology as an applied profession is being delivered in more diverse ways. One avenue for doing this is through community, voluntary, and social enterprises (CVSEs) (Kapadia et al., 2022; Rachael 2011). This enables neuropsychology to be accessible to people from disadvantaged backgrounds whilst simultaneously challenging the view of neuropsychology as a White-only profession. Just Psychology (Fatimilehin et al., 2015) and INSneuro CIC are two social enterprise organisations doing just that. As a contribution to workforce development and diversification, INSneuro CIC runs an aspiring psychologist programme. This supports and mentors aspiring neuropsychologists, particularly those most disadvantaged due to ethnicity and social inequalities. Community organisations serving minoritised ethnic communities also have access to neuropsychology training, interventions, and consultation. It is recommended that clinical neuropsychology service providers actively collaborate with community organisations to co-produce services and diversify the neuropsychology workforce. This is one way to increase the reach, impact, and effectiveness with more marginalised communities.

Conclusion

The neurorehabilitation setting is a microcosm of intersecting cultures (Uomoto, 2016). Despite this, when discussing and applying the principles of multicultural neuropsychology, we cannot assume that the workforce has a shared understanding and acceptance of this. However, as clinical neuropsychologists, we must ensure that we have invested the time and effort needed to become more culturally aware and culturally sensitive. We also have a unique opportunity to create spaces within clinical neuropsychology to examine ourselves, individually and collectively, as a profession and address some of the difficult and distressing issues that may emerge.

References

Adetimole, F., Afuape, T., & Vara, V. (2005). The impact of racism on the experience of training on a clinical psychology course: Reflections from three black trainees. *Clinical Psychology Forum, 48*, 11–15.

Ashan, S. (2022, April). EDI: Endless Distraction and Inaction. *The Psychologist*, 22–26.

Baber, Z. (2020). *An exploration of the perspectives of neuropsychologists working with clients from ethnically, culturally and linguistically diverse background.* (ProfDoc Thesis, University of East London), 29. Retrieved from https://repository.uel.ac.uk/item/8886.

BPS. (2020). EDI Taskforce. *British Psychological Society.* Retrieved from https://BPS.org.uk/about-us/diversity-and-inclusion/taskforce.

BPS. (2021). *BPS Strategic Framework 2021–22.* BPS Publications.

Clearing House for Postgraduate Course in Clinical Psychology. (2021). Places by Course Centre – 2020 Entry. *Clearing House for Postgraduate Courses in Clinical Psychology.* Retrieved from https://www.leeds.ac.uk/chpccp/numbersplaces2020.pdf.

Fatimilehin, I., Pilkington, A., van Silfhout, K., & McCann, M. (2015). Developing a cultural consultancy service. *Clinical Psychology Forum, 273*, 24–28.

Hays, P. A. (2016). *Addressing Cultural Complexities in Practice: Assessment, diagnosis and therapy* (3rd ed.). American Psychological Association. Retrieved from https:/doi.org/10.1037/14801-000.

Health Education England. (2021). *Psychological Professions Workforce Plan for England.* NHS: Health Education England: Psychological Professions, 6.

Kapadia, D., Zhang, J., Salway, S., Nazroo, J., Booth, A., Villarroel-Williams, N., Bècares, L., & Esmail, A. (2022). *Ethnic Inequalities in Healthcare: A rapid evidence review.* NHS Race & Health Observatory.

Kline, R. (2021). *No More Tick Boxes: A review of the evidence on how to make recruitment and career progression fairer.* NHS East of England.

Likupe, G., & Archibong, U. (2013). Black African Nurses' Experiences of Equality, Racism, and Discrimination in the National Health Service. *Journal of Psychological Issues in Organizational Culture, 3*(S1), 227–246. DOI: 10.1002/JPOC.21071.

Nugent, L. (2019). Whiteness and clinical psychology: Acknowledging its presence and role on perpetuating racist trauma. *Clinical Psychology Forum, 319,* 12–14.

Odusanya, S. O. E., Winter, D., Nolte, L., & Shah, S. (2018). The Experience of Being a Qualified Female BME Clinical Psychologist in a National Health Service: An Interpretative Phenomenological and Repertory Grid Analysis. *Journal of Constructivist Psychology, 31*(3), 273–291. DOI: 10.1080/10720537.2017.1304301.

Onyeama, F., & Yates-Stephenson, N. (2020, October 27). Harsh truths on the clinical journey. *The Psychologist.* Retrieved from https://thepsychologist.bps.org.uk/harsh-truths-clinical-journey.

Palmer, W., Schlepper, L., Hemmings, N., & Crellin, N. (2021). *The right track: Participation and progression in psychology career pathways,* 11. Nuffield Trust.

Rachael, A. (2011). *Social Enterprise in Health Care.* The Kings Fund.

Rajan, L., & Shaw, S. K. (2008). 'I can only speak for myself': Some voices from black and minority ethnic clinical psychology trainees. *Clinical Psychology Forum, 190,* 11–16.

Rhead, R. D., Chui, Z., Bakolis I., ... & Hatch, S. L. (2021). Impact of workplace discrimination and harassment among National Health Service staff working in London trusts: Results from the TIDES study. *British Journal of Psychology Open Access, 7*(1), e10. DOI: 10.1192/BJO.2020.137.

Ross, S., Jabbal, J., Chauhan, K., Maguire, D., Randawa, M., & Dahir, S. (2020). *Workforce race inequality and inclusion in NHS providers*. The King's Fund.

Uomoto, J. (2016). *Multicultural neurorehabilitation: Clinical principles for rehabilitation professionals*. Preface. Springer Publications.

Workforce Race Equality Standard. (2021). *NHS Workforce Race Equality Standard: 2020 Data Analysis Report for NHS Trusts and Clinical Commissioning Groups*. NHS WRES.

Yates, P. (2017). DoN membership survey and membership network demographics. *The Neuropsychologist, 3*.

14 Future Directions in Neuropsychology and Concluding Comments

Ndidi Boakye and Amanda Mwale

Our ability to reach unity in diversity will be the beauty and the test of our civilization.

Mahatma Gandhi

As we reflect on Gandhi's words above, we cannot help but marvel that they still ring true some 50-odd years since they were uttered. We are still grappling as a society to reach unity in our diversity, but perhaps the focus of the journey is not the destination but the desire to continue to reach that goal. We must strive to do the necessary work of reflecting on our current processes, examining ourselves and our clinical practices, and adapting practices to meet the needs of a range of individuals, families, and communities.

As co-authors and co-editors, we recognise that we share minoritised characteristics: we are Black African, Christian, cisgendered females from Nigerian and Zimbabwean ancestry respectively. In reflecting on the process of putting this book together, our joint experiences of witnessing and experiencing bias have stirred up our commitment to progress and change.

This book began by proposing the idea of multicultural neuropsychology, a hopeful start in embedding cultural perspectives into effective rehabilitation practices. In recent years, the knowledge and awareness surrounding health inequalities have increased, no doubt advanced by the COVID-19 pandemic. However, there is remarkably little written about cultural disparities within the UK neurorehabilitation literature. As a profession, neuropsychologists discuss these issues; however, there is a focus on the assessment process (Fernández & Abe, 2017; Fernández & Evans, 2022). Since the COVID-19 pandemic, there has been some examination of who accesses neuropsychology services (Dunning & Teager, 2020). There has also been a call for more inclusive practices within neuropsychology (Division of Neuropsychology, 2021). We hope that the recommendations highlighted in the 'Multicultural Neuropsychology' chapter (Chapter 1) is a starting point in addressing some of this. The offer of a new, adapted formulation model that goes beyond

DOI: 10.4324/9781003309819-19

the traditional boundaries of the biopsychosocial model by emphasising the role of social and cultural contexts in shaping problems is welcomed. Furthermore, the need for interventions to go beyond the individual in the therapy room is stressed. This is not a panacea but the foundation of work that future research and interventions can be built on.

We value the guidance offered in the chapters 'Navigating Intersectionality in Couple Therapy for Brain Injury' (Chapter 4) and 'Good Teams Mind Their GGRRAAACCEEESSS' (Chapter 2). The importance of developing a shared understanding as a clinical team when working with patients is crucial. The link between the team formulation and patient care has long been established (Holmes, 2002; Kerr, Dent-Brown, & Parry, 2007), and the ability for a team to explore the impact of social and contextual factors on patient care cannot be underestimated. We are hopeful that the reflective practice models highlighted will offer contained and safe ways in which shared formulations can be developed in the neurorehabilitation context. This will facilitate the adjustment process for individuals and families living with brain injury. Adjustment is part of the process that underpins the formation of identity in the context of brain injury. In our clinical practice, we recognised that using the narrative-therapy-informed 'Tree of Life' approach in brain injury (Chapter 3) can support reconnecting individuals and families with their history, culture, values, loved ones, skills, contributions, hopes, and dreams. It is our hope that this will support in further thickening their preferred stories and identities.

We are facing a time of change globally in the way difference is viewed by society. In paediatric neurorehabilitation, attention is being given to greater integration, cross-departmental working, and the need to recognise the often hidden and invisible nature of ABI. The authors of Chapter 5 identified that this brings opportunities for action. They name the strengths and limitations in current service delivery and the bias within the foundations upon which 'evidence-led' practice is based. We welcome new approaches and developments that will take place within the paediatric professional literature.

We couldn't pull together a book in the digital age without giving some consideration to technology and its clinical application. We hope you will be as inspired as we were to read about Dr. Trayner's innovative practices and how they contribute to levelling access to neurorehabilitation (Chapter 9). We repeat her call for clinicians to get involved in the use of technology to innovate and to streamline our clinical processes so we can make real progress in accessibility even in the absence of an increase in the availability of services or funding.

There is much meat on the bone in the wealth of clinical experiences shared in this book addressing inclusion in clinical practice. Dr. Ehsan (Chapter 6) shares valuable insights in how to lessen the likelihood of bias when conducting neuropsychological assessment, whilst Dr. Berry-Khan

(Chapter 7) explores these considerations in personal injury work. The discussions about the impact of microaggressions on well-being, engagement, and clinical care is timely, as are the refreshing insights offered by Dr. Agnew (Chapter 10) when queering neuropsychology. Dr. Agnew's ideas are somewhat pioneering in the UK context, and we look forward to others building on the foundations he lays.

However, none of this work can take place without good leadership. Dr. Mobley (Chapter 12) and Drs. Haye, Sundin, and Rahim (Chapter 11) write eloquently about leadership at different stages of the professional trajectory and the teaching of new 'generations' of professionals. Dr. Sampson (Chapter 13) takes these ideas further in her reminder that the neurorehabilitation setting is a microcosm of intersecting cultures (Uomoto, 2016). She stresses that, as clinical neuropsychologists, we must ensure that we have invested the time and effort needed to become more culturally aware and culturally sensitive. This starts with looking at our workforce and recruitment processes.

Finally, it is important to state that we did not cover every aspect of identity, nor do we wish to position ourselves as the all-knowing 'experts' in this area. We are committed to continuing our learning, and in this book we have offered a collection of our own clinical experiences and insights. These have addressed intersectionality and our attempts to provide a path for greater inclusivity in the context of neurorehabilitation. In order to continue to lay the foundations and take this work further, it is essential that more skilled clinicians come forward to support the evolution of equitable practices. There is a need for research in the area – for example, microaggressions in neurorehabilitation (Chapter 8) as well as vocational and clinical outcomes for different ethnic groups, including other minoritised subgroups within those communities. There is much to be explored, including biases in team formulation and the impact on patients' trajectory of care and clinical outcomes. There is a need for examination of supervision, training, and recruitment practices and their role in maintaining bias in the current workforce. It is our shared responsibility to ensure that every individual that comes into contact with our neurorehabilitation services is welcomed and treated with dignity, respect, and equity. Therefore, we end by inviting you and your colleagues to join us in continuing this work in solidarity.

References

Division of Neuropsychology. (2021, October 14–15). Equality, Diversity & Inclusion in Clinical Neuropsychology: Committing to Action. Division of Neuropsychology Conference 2021, British Psychological Society, online.

Dunning, G., & Teager, A. (2020). An evaluation of ethnicity in a neuropsychology outpatient department. Division of Clinical Psychology (DCP) Annual Conference: Doing What Matters: Value-Driven Clinical Psychology in Action.

Fernández, A. L., & Abe, J. (2017). Bias in cross-cultural neuropsychological testing: Problems and possible solutions. *Culture and Brain, 6*(1), 1–35.

Fernández, A. L., & Evans, J. (Eds.). (2022). *Understanding Cross-cultural Neuropsychology: Science, Testing and Challenges.* Routledge.

Holmes, J. (2002). Acute wards: Problems and solutions: Creating a psychotherapeutic culture in acute psychiatric wards. *Psychiatric Bulletin, 26*(10), 383–385.

Kerr, I. B., Dent-Brown, K., & Parry, G. D. (2007). Psychotherapy and mental health teams. *International Review of Psychiatry, 19*(1), 63–80.

Uotomo, J. (2016). *Multicultural neurorehabilitation: Clinical principles for rehabilitation professionals.* Springer Publications.

Afterword

Fergus Gracey

Clinical Associate Professor in Clinical Psychology,
Norwich Medical School

This pioneering volume presents for the first time a UK perspective on addressing equality and inclusion in various domains in neuropsychological practice. The book emphasises what is at stake (in terms of oppressive practice, micro aggressions, dehumanisation, the right to equitable healthcare) if we fail to proactively bring the focus on minoritised groups and related intersectionality front and centre in our practice. The chapters raise awareness of the research which unarguably maps the historical and current inequalities in the profession of clinical neuropsychology in terms of workforce, equality of service provision, and the multiple aspects of neuropsychological assessment and intervention that perpetuate oppression and injustice to those not from a White, Eurocentric, and heteronormative background. This makes for uncomfortable reading, holding attention to the shocking failings of our profession. At the same time, the authors bring to attention innovative concepts and practices across multiple contexts responding to the systems, structures, and types of diversity in our UK communities. In this sense the discomfort of historical and current injustice is to an extent offset by practical ideas for evolving practice and an overarching message of inspiration and hope for change.

So, that is my general summary of the content of the book. However, for me, reading this book has taken me beyond simply reflecting on the information content and the useful ideas for innovative practice. It prompts me to reflect deeply on my current and past work and my own personal life: on the work I have written about and shared publicly; on my clinical and leadership roles; and on my work as a lecturer, advisor, and research supervisor to trainee clinical psychologists. I look back with a sense of shame at the times I have not been open or attentive to aspects of difference in my clinical work. I can readily see moments where I have fallen short of what was needed to be inclusive, to be sensitive to the contexts people have brought to interactions with me. And I notice my reaction, the discomfort, and the urge to respond: 'It seems I have unwittingly [insert act of White oppression here]'. And why do I want to say 'seems' and 'unwittingly'? Why the compulsion to remove my 'self' from these occasions?

I also reflect on my own life experiences; my complex relationships with my class, nationality, and especially gender; personal experiences of exclusion and othering; involvement in activism ... and realise again that this is not enough. We all have our contexts, our histories, our complexities, and the simple fact of this is not enough to ensure that we will necessarily understand and be sensitive to the contexts and circumstances of others without consciously and concertedly doing so. So, I hold for a moment and stay with the shame, the confusion, and reflect more on that and further gut reactions towards apology, humility, activism ... but again I try to stop and sit with this knot of emotion, acknowledge this, and consider more carefully the actions I now need to take.

Thinking about the things I have written about in my career, the concepts I have promoted, and in doing so the issues I have neglected or turned away from, there's a dizzying realisation of the extent of the problem we are facing – a kind of vertigo looking at the depths to which the 'status quo' in our profession is problematic. We have as a profession in recent times begun the unravelling process, but to hasten this now I will need to bring more consciousness to practice in clinical psychology training and research, especially. Why are we researching *this* topic, why are we promoting *this* concept as important and valid, why is *this* perspective dominant in our thinking? And what are the consequences of these ideas for those not from a White, heteronormative background and for building a truly inclusive and humanising profession? Alongside this, I will need to attend with greater openness and curiosity to interactions with others, especially those from minoritized backgrounds and, as a general principle, to 'assume nothing and question everything'. And I can see that this is only a start, a shifting of the conceptual landscape that might make improvements to inclusivity possible. But, as a wider profession, we will also need to keep engaging with the facts of oppressive practice, reflecting and talking to make sure there are safe spaces for us to all engage with the horror of what has gone before and process this in a constructive way so as to take actions in our everyday practice that authentically and deeply change things for the better.

To help us along on this journey, this pioneering volume provides us with some key examples of practice development from assessment to intervention with adults and children, indirect working with teams, service models, and workforce planning across public sector and private, acute, and community settings. There is no doubt that issues of inequality and oppression reverberate across all of these domains, and with this book the authors, under the studied guidance of Boakye and Mwale, lay the foundations for a hopeful revolution in UK clinical neuropsychology practice that will indeed challenge the status quo.

Index

Note: **Bold** page numbers refer to tables, *italic* page numbers refer to figures.

For Product Safety Concerns and Information please contact our EU
representative GPSR@taylorandfrancis.com
Taylor & Francis Verlag GmbH, Kaufingerstraße 24, 80331 München, Germany